Neuroendovascular Management: Anatomy and Techniques

Guest Editors

ROBERT H. ROSENWASSER, MD, FACS, FAHA
PASCAL M. JABBOUR, MD

NEUROSURGERY CLINICS OF NORTH AMERICA

www.neurosurgery.theclinics.com

Consulting Editors

ANDREW T. PARSA, MD, PhD
PAUL C. McCORMICK, MD, MPH

July 2009 • Volume 20 • Number 3

SAUNDERS an imprint of ELSEVIER, Inc.

W.B. SAUNDERS COMPANY
A Division of Elsevier Inc.

1600 John F. Kennedy Blvd. • Suite 1800 • Philadelphia, PA 19103-2899

http://www.theclinics.com

NEUROSURGERY CLINICS OF NORTH AMERICA Volume 20, Number 3
July 2009 ISSN 1042-3680, ISBN-13: 978-1-4377-0507-2, ISBN-10: 1-4377-0507-3

Editor: Joanne Husovski
Developmental Editor: Donald Mumford

Neurosurgery Clinics of North America (ISSN 1042-3680) is published quarterly by Elsevier Inc., 360 Park Avenue South, New York, NY 10010-1710. Months of issue are January, April, July, and October. Business and Editorial Offices: 1600 John F. Kennedy Blvd., Suite 1800, Philadelphia, PA 19103-2899. Customer Service Office: 11830 Westline Industrial Drive, St. Louis, MO 63146. Periodicals postage paid at New York, NY, and additional mailing offices. Subscription prices are $274.00 per year (US individuals), $438.00 per year (US institutions), $300.00 per year (Canadian individuals), $535.00 per year (Canadian institutions), $383.00 per year (international individuals), $535.00 per year (international institutions), $138.00 per year (US students), and $189.00 per year (international students). International air speed delivery is included in all *Clinics* subscription prices. All prices are subject to change without notice. **POSTMASTER:** Send address changes to *Neurosurgery Clinics of North America*, Elsevier Periodicals Customer Service, 11830 Westline Industrial Drive, St. Louis, MO 63146. **Customer Service: 1-800-654-2452 (US and Canada). From outside the US and Canada, call: 1-314-453-7041. Fax: 1-314-453-5170.** E-mail: JournalsCustomerService-usa@elsevier.com **(for print support) and** journalsonlinesupport-usa@elsevier.com **(for online support).**

Reprints. For copies of 100 or more, of articles in this publication, please contact the Commercial Reprints Department, Elsevier Inc., 360 Park Avenue South, New York, NY 10010-1710. Tel. (212) 633-3812; Fax: (212) 462-1935; E-mail: reprints@elsevier.com.

Neurosurgery Clinics of North America is covered in *MEDLINE/PubMed (Index Medicus), EMBASE/Excerpta Medica, and Current Contents/Clinical Medicine (CC/CM).*

Contributors

GUEST EDITORS

ROBERT H. ROSENWASSER, MD, FACS, FAHA
Professor and Chairman, Department of Neurological Surgery; Professor of Radiology, Thomas Jefferson University, Philadelphia, Pennsylvania

PASCAL M. JABBOUR, MD
Assistant Professor of Neurological Surgery, Thomas Jefferson University, Philadelphia, Pennsylvania

AUTHORS

ROCCO A. ARMONDA, MC, USA
Director of Cerebrovascular Neurosurgery and Interventional Neuroradiology, Department of Neurosurgery, National Capital Consortium, Walter Reed Army Medical Center, Washington, DC; Department of Neurosurgery, National Capital Consortium, National Naval Medical Center, Bethesda, Maryland

TIBOR BECSKE, MD
Department of Neurology; Department of Neurosurgery; Department of Radiology, New York University, Langone Medical Center, New York

RANDY BELL, MC, USN
Neurovascular Fellow, Departments of Neurosurgery and Neuroradiology, Washington Hospital Center, Washington, DC; Staff Neurosurgeon, Department of Neurosurgery, National Naval Medical Center; Assistant Professor, Department of Neurosurgery, Uniformed Services University of the Health Sciences, Bethesda, Maryland

BERNARD R. BENDOK, MD
Endovascular Surgical Neuroradiology, Department of Neurosurgery; Division of Neuroradiology, Department of Radiology, Northwestern University Feinberg School of Medicine, Chicago, Illinois

N. CHAUDHARY
Neuroendovascular Fellow, Department of Radiology/Neuroradiology, University of Michigan Hospitals, Ann Arbor, Michigan

PENG R. CHEN, MD
Department of Neurosurgery, University of Texas at Houston, Houston, Texas

GUILHERME DABUS, MD
Department of Neurosurgery; Division of Neuroradiology, Department of Radiology, Northwestern University Feinberg School of Medicine, Chicago, Illinois

MICHAEL L. DILUNA, MD
Department of Neurosurgery, Yale University School of Medicine, New Haven, Connecticut

RICHARD G. FESSLER, MD
Department of Neurosurgery, Northwestern University Feinberg School of Medicine, Chicago, Illinois

J.J. GEMMETE
Assistant Professor, Department of Radiology/Neuroradiology, University of Michigan Hospitals, Ann Arbor, Michigan

RICHARD J.T. GORNIAK, MD
Assistant Professor of Radiology, Division of Neuroradiology, Department of Radiology, Thomas Jefferson University and Hospital, Philadelphia, Pennsylvania

MICHAEL B. HOROWITZ, MD
Departments of Neurological Surgery and
Radiology, University of Pittsburgh Medical
Center, Pittsburgh, Pennsylvania

MICHAEL C. HURLEY, MD
Endovascular Surgical Neuroradiology
Department of Neurosurgery; Division
of Neuroradiology, Department
of Radiology, Northwestern University
Feinberg School of Medicine, Chicago,
Illinois

MICHELE H. JOHNSON, MD
Associate Professor Diagnostic Radiology,
Surgery (Otolaryngology) and Neurosurgery
Director, Interventional Neuroradiology, Yale
University School of Medicine, New Haven,
Connecticut

RAMI KAAKAJI, MD
Division of Neuroradiology, Department of
Radiology, Northwestern University Feinberg
School of Medicine, Chicago, Illinois

KENNETH M. LIEBMAN, MD, FACS
Stroke and Cerebrovascular Center of New
Jersey, Capital Health System, Hamilton,
New Jersey

PETER KIM NELSON, MD
Associate Professor, Department of Radiology;
Department of Neurosurgery, New York
University, Langone Medical Center,
New York, New York

A.S. PANDEY
Assistant Professor, Department
of Neurosurgery, University of Michigan,
Ann Arbor, Michigan

ALI SHAIBANI, MD
Department of Neurosurgery; Division of
Neuroradiology, Department of Radiology,
Northwestern University Feinberg School of
Medicine, Chicago, Illinois

MERYL A. SEVERSON III, MC, USN
Staff Neurosurgeon, Department of
Neurosurgery, National Capital Consortium,
Walter Reed Army Medical Center,
Washington, DC; Department
of Neurosurgery, National Capital
Consortium, National Naval Medical Center,
Bethesda, Maryland

ADNAN H. SIDDIQUI, MD, PhD
Department of Neurosurgery, School of
Medicine and Biomedical Sciences, Millard
Fillmore Gates Hospital, Kaleida Health, State
University of New York, University at Buffalo,
Buffalo, New York

LISA M. TARTAGLINO, MD
Associate Professor of Radiology, Division
of Neuroradiology, Department of Radiology,
Thomas Jefferson University and Hospital,
Philadelphia, Pennsylvania

B.G. THOMPSON, MD
Professor of Neurosurgery, Department
of Neurosurgery, University of Michigan,
Ann Arbor, Michigan

HJALTI M. THORRISON, MD
Attending Radiologist, Department of
Radiology, University Hospital of Iceland,
Reykjavik, Iceland; Adjunct Assistant
Professor, Yale University School of Medicine,
New Haven, Connecticut

NESTOR D. TOMYCZ, MD
Departments of Neurological Surgery and
Radiology, University of Pittsburgh Medical
Center, Pittsburgh, Pennsylvania

MATHEW T. WALKER, MD
Division of Neuroradiology, Department
of Radiology, Northwestern University
Feinberg School of Medicine, Chicago,
Illinois

Contents

Because no single test is definitive for Cushing's disease (CD), establishing the diagnosis has remained a challenge that relies on building a critical mass of evidence. The differential diagnosis of corticotropin (ACTH)-dependent Cushing's syndrome (CS) traditionally has rested on noninvasive biochemical and radiologic testing. Bilateral inferior petrosal sinus sampling (BIPSS) is an invasive procedure that has become part of the diagnostic armamentarium surrounding CD. When used appropriately—that is, for patients who have biochemically confirmed ACTH-dependent CS but discordant biochemical or radiologic studies—BIPSS is the reference standard confirmatory test for CD.

The balloon test occlusion is one method by which surgeons evaluate whether a patient will be able to tolerate permanent occlusion of an extracranial or intracranial vessel. This article discusses the indications, methods, predictive value, and complications of the balloon test occlusion. It also briefly describes the Wada test in the context of preoperative evaluation of patients who are candidates for temporal lobectomy.

Neurosurgery Clinics of North America

THE CLINICS ARE NOW AVAILABLE ONLINE!

Access your subscription at:
www.theclinics.com

Preface

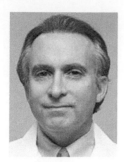 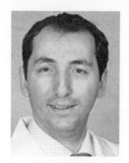

Robert H. Rosenwasser, MD, FACS, FAHA   Pascal M. Jabbour, MD
Guest Editors

This is the first of two issues on a series of current thoughts, concepts, and practice of neuroendovascular therapy.

The authors of these two issues come from backgrounds in neurology, neurosurgery, and interventional neuroradiology, demonstrating the way in which the various disciplines have come together for better patient care.

Issue I deals with concepts of neurovascular anatomy of the head, neck, and skull base and with practical approaches to certain anatomical variables. Sections on imaging using CT, magnetic resonance, and ultrasound have also been included as they apply to neuroendovascular procedures. The issue concludes with an article on a time-proven method preceding a deconstructive procedure dealing with balloon occlusion tests.

The authors of these two issues are thought leaders in the field and have contributed a great deal. We feel certain that you will find these two issues timely and informative. They will undoubtedly be the mainstay of references for some time to come.

I wish to acknowledge all the authors for their diligence and effort in preparing their contributions for these two issues.

Robert H. Rosenwasser, MD, FACS, FAHA
Professor and Chairman
Department of Neurological Surgery
Professor of Radiology
Thomas Jefferson University
909 Walnut Street, 3rd Floor
Philadelphia, PA 19107, USA

Pascal M. Jabbour, MD
Assistant Professor of Neurological Surgery
Thomas Jefferson University
909 Walnut Street, 3rd Floor
Philadelphia, PA 19107, USA

E-mail addresses:
Robert.Rosenwasser@Jefferson.edu
(R.H. Rosenwasser)
pascal.jabbour@jefferson.edu (P.M. Jabbour)

doi:10.1016/j.nec.2009.07.002
1042-3680/09/$ – see front matter

neurosurgery.theclinics.com

Vascular Anatomy: The Head, Neck, and Skull Base

Michele H. Johnson, MD[a],*, Hjalti M. Thorisson, MD[b,c],
Michael L. DiLuna, MD[d]

KEYWORDS

- Cervical-cerebral anatomy • Aortic arch
- Collateral pathways • Vertebral artery
- Carotid arteries • Extracranial • Vascular anastomoses

The vasculature of the head and neck, beginning with the origins of the great vessels at the aortic arch and extending through the skull base, can be thought of as "a vascular highway." The vessels traverse and supply important soft tissue and bony structures. Vascular displacements, anomalous or congenital variations, susceptibility to vascular injury, and neovascular supply to mass lesions are all "sights we see along the way." Our purpose is to highlight the normal anatomic features, and common and uncommon vascular variants that may affect cross-sectional image analysis and angiographic diagnosis, thus impacting therapeutic management.[1,2]

AORTIC ARCH AND BRANCHES

The aorta emerges from the pericardium of the heart and proceeds within the superior mediastinum to form the ascending aortic arch, and lies anterior to the trachea at the level of the sternal manubrium. From the ascending arch, embryologically formed from the left fourth primitive aortic arch, arise 3 major branches (from proximal to distal): the innominate or brachiocephalic artery (BCA), the left common carotid artery (LCCA), and the left subclavian artery (LSUB) (**Fig. 1**A).[3–7]

The BCA ascends obliquely cephalad and toward the right, anterior to the trachea before bifurcating into the right common carotid and right subclavian artery (RSUB) behind the sternoclavicular joint. Fluoroscopically, the head of the clavicle marks the location of the bifurcation of the BCA and can be a useful adjunct to selective catheterization. Turning the patient's head toward the left and extending the right arm accentuates the separation between the anteriorly located right common carotid artery (RCCA) and the more posteriorly located RSUB and straightens the course of the RSUB facilitating catheterization. In approximately 20% of patients the LCCA arises in conjunction with the BCA, referred to as a bovine configuration (**Fig. 1**B).[8,9] The left vertebral artery may arise directly from the aortic arch in 5% of cases, and it is often smaller in caliber (**Fig. 1**C). Rarely there may be dual left vertebral supply with a branch of the subclavian artery joining the left vertebral artery arising from the aortic arch just before the vertebral artery entry into the foramen transversarium. The right vertebral artery may also rarely arise directly from the aortic arch.[10] An aberrant RSUB is an aortic arch variation whereby the aberrant RSUB arises as the distal-most branch from the aortic arch, and

[a] Department of Diagnostic Radiology, Interventional Neuroradiology, Yale University School of Medicine, 333 Cedar Street, PO Box 8082, New Haven, CT 06520, USA
[b] Department of Radiology, University Hospital—Landspitali Haskolasjukrahus i Fossvogi, University Hospital of Iceland, Reykjavik, Iceland
[c] Department of Diagnostic Radiology, Yale University School of Medicine, 333 Cedar Street, PO Box 8082, New Haven, CT 06520, USA
[d] Department of Neurosurgery, Yale University School of Medicine, 333 Cedar Street, PO Box 8082, New Haven, CT 06520, USA
* Corresponding author.
E-mail address: michele.h.johnson@yale.edu (M.H. Johnson).

Neurosurg Clin N Am 20 (2009) 239–258
doi:10.1016/j.nec.2009.07.001
1042-3680/09/$ – see front matter © 2009 Published by Elsevier Inc.

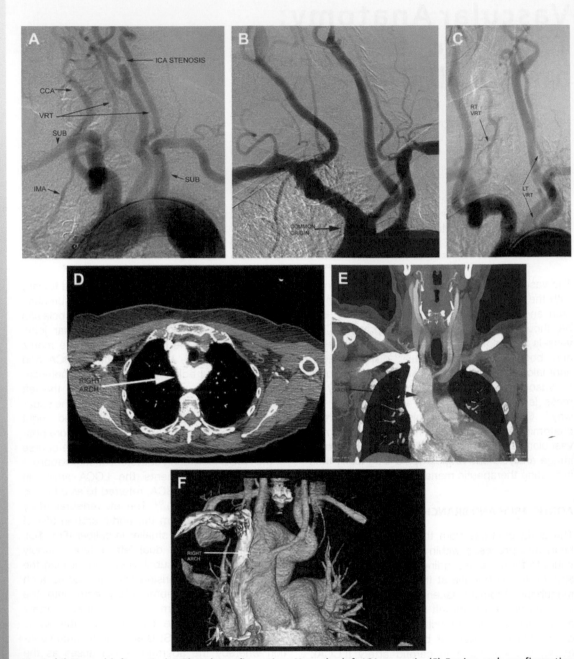

Fig. 1. (*A*) Normal left aortic (LAO) arch configuration. Note the left ICA stenosis. (*B*) Bovine arch configuration is demonstrated with a common origin of the innominate artery and the left CCA. (*C*) Left vertebral artery (VRT) arises from the aortic arch between the origins of the left CCA and the left subclavian artery (SUB). (*D*) to (*F*) Mirror image right aortic arch. Axial computed tomographic angiography (CTA) image (*D*) demonstrates the right aortic arch that is clearly demonstrated on the coronal reformatted maximum intensity projection (MIP) image (*E*). The three-dimensional reformatted image (*F*) demonstrates the mirror image orientation of the arch.

proceeds toward the right behind the esophagus, to give rise to the right vertebral artery and the remaining subclavian artery branches. In such a case, the RCCA arises as the first branch from the aortic arch followed by the LCCA, the LSUB, and then the RSUB The aorta adjacent to the origin of the aberrant right subclavian may be focally dilated, referred to as a Kommerell diverticulum, and may become aneurysmal, requiring surgical repair or diversion (**Fig. 1**D, E).[11,12]

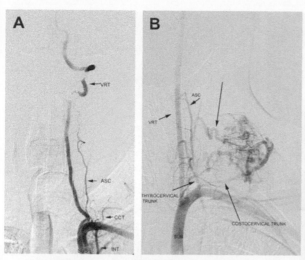

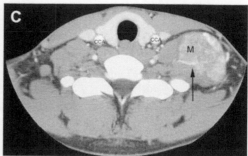

Fig. 2. (*A*) Anteroposterior (AP) subclavian arteriogram demonstrates a normal appearance of the cervical portion of the vertebral artery (VRT), the ascending cervical artery (ASC), the internal mammary artery (IMT) and the costocervical trunk (CCT). (*B*) AP subclavian arteriogram in a patient with a supraclavicular pulsatile mass demonstrates neovascularity derived from branches of the thyrocervical (TCT) and costocervical trunks. (*C*) Contrast CT scan demonstrates the vessels traversing the mass which was biopsy-proven hemangioma.

SUBCLAVIAN AND VERTEBRAL ARTERIES

The vertebral arteries arise from the subclavian arteries from the posterosuperior wall, just opposite the origin of the internal mammary artery. Additional important subclavian branches include the thyrocervical trunk, the ascending cervical artery, and costocervical trunks (**Fig. 2**A–C).[1,5,6] The thyrocervical trunk contributes flow to the anterior aspect of the thyroid gland and adjacent musculature. The ascending cervical artery provides supply to the posterior cervical musculature but also represents a significant source of collateral flow in the setting of vertebral artery occlusion usually joining the native vertebral artery at the level of C3 (**Fig. 3**). The costocervical trunk also supplies blood to the cervical musculature and brachial plexus. The subclavian branches are important to analyze with respect to pathologic processes of the lower neck, such as vascular

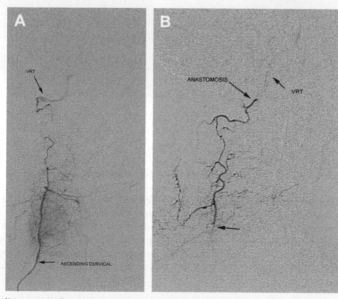

Fig. 3. Selective ascending cervical arteriogram demonstrates anastomosis with the vertebral artery (VRT) at the level of C3 on AP (*A*) and lateral (*B*) views.

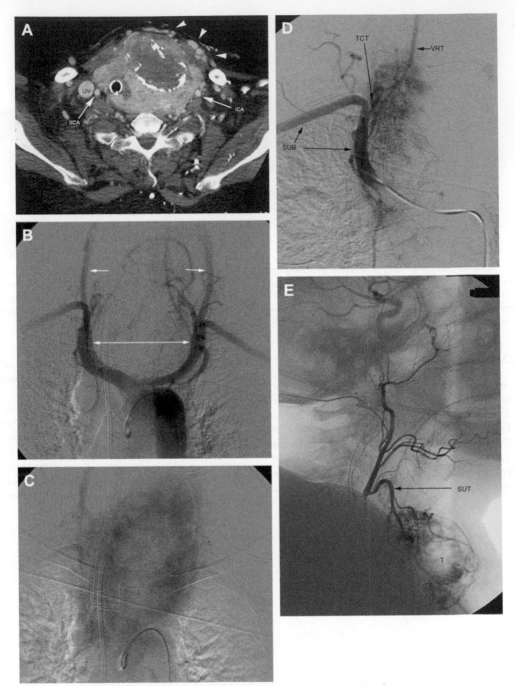

Fig. 4. (*A*) Contrast-enhanced axial CT scan demonstrates a large heterogeneous mass arising from the thyroid with central necrosis and calcification. Note the displacement of the trachea toward the right and enlargement of multiple dilated venous collaterals (arrowheads) anterior to the mass in the setting of left internal jugular and superior vena caval obstruction. Note the displacement of the CCAs which are splayed by the intervening mass. Early (*B*) and late (*C*) images from the arch arteriogram confirm the splaying of the CCA and demonstrate an intense vascular blush consistent with the biopsy diagnosis of thyroid carcinoma. (*D*) RSUB injection reveals an intense neovascular blush derived from branches of the thyrocervical trunk and ascending cervical arteries. (*E*) Right common carotid injection demonstrates a similar neovascular blush from the superior thyroid artery.

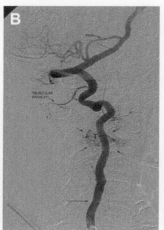
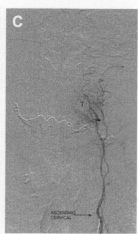
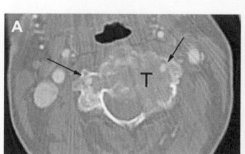

Fig. 5. (A) Axial CTA image demonstrates the expansile and destructive mass (T) involving the C2 vertebra with encroachment on both vertebral arteries, right > left. (B) Selective right vertebral injection demonstrates mild neovascularity arising from vertebral body branches of the vertebral artery. (C) AP selective injection of the ascending cervical artery shows additional neovascularity and a distal communication to the vertebral artery, precluding preoperative embolization. Surgical pathology revealed metastatic lung cancer.

malformations and masses involving the soft tissue neck and cervical or upper thoracic vertebral bodies and spinal cord (Fig. 4).

The vertebral arteries course posterior to the common carotid arteries beneath the longus coli and scalenus anterior muscles and enter the transverse foramen at approximately C6. They traverse the transverse foramen between C6 and proceed posterolateral to C2 and then ascend posteromedially between C1 and the occiput before piercing the dura as they enter the foramen magnum.[1,5,6] The cervical portion of the vertebral artery provides branches to the normal vertebral bodies and the adjacent cervical musculature, as well as providing supply to the metastatic and primary bone and soft tissue tumors (Fig. 5). The cervical vertebral course is usually straight although tortuosity, including significant loops, may occur and cause confusion in the setting of trauma or tumor. It should be

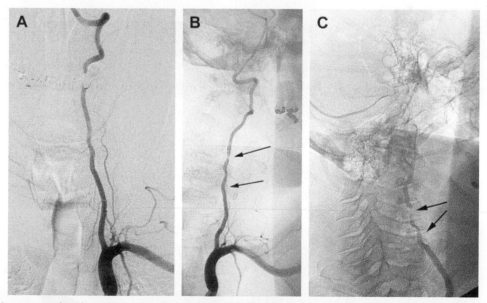

Fig. 6. Syncope on head turning. (A) Left vertebral artery, neutral position. Note the compression of the cervical vertebral artery by uncovertebral joint degenerative osteophytes accentuated on moderate (B) and maximal (C) head turning. (From Johnson et al. Vascular anatomy of the head, neck, and skull base. In Hurst RW, Rosenwasser RH, editors. Interventional neuroradiology. New York: Taylor and Frances; 2007; with permission.)

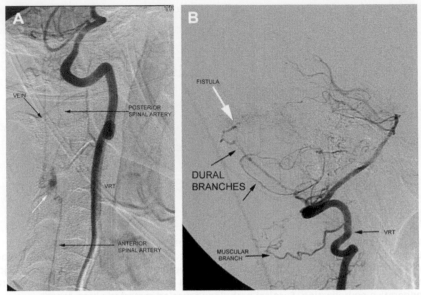

Fig. 7. (*A*) Lateral view from a vertebral artery (VRT) injection demonstrates the anterior and posterior spinal vertebral branches supplying the neovascular supply to a spinal hemangioblastoma. (*B*) Lateral upper cervical and intracranial vertebral artery angiogram shows the different appearance and courses of the straight dural branches, the undulating muscular branches and the pial branches of the vertebral artery in this patient with a dural arteriovenous malformation (fistula).

noted that luminal narrowing or compromise may occur with head turning and may be accentuated by the presence of osteophytes which may encroach on the artery within the transverse foramen (**Fig. 6**).[2,13] Provocative maneuvers such as head turning during angiography or during cross-sectional imaging may be of value

in demonstrating such narrowing that may correlate with clinical hypoperfusion syndromes.[13–15] Anastomoses exist at multiple cervical levels with the external carotid artery (ECA) branches, the thyrocervical trunk, the costocervical trunk, and ascending cervical arteries (see **Fig. 5**). The concept of vertebral artery dominance relates to

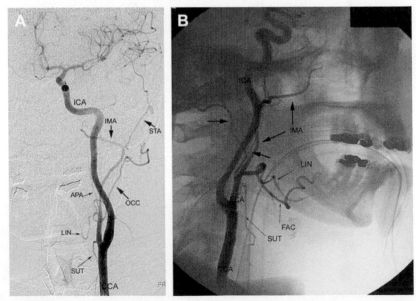

Fig. 8. (*A*) AP and (*B*) lateral views of 2 different patients on common carotid injections showing the branching pattern of the ECA and the typical common and internal carotid course. (IMA, internal maxillary; STA, superficial temporal; OCC, occipital; APA, ascending pharyngeal; LIN, lingual; FAC, facial; SUT, superior thyroid).

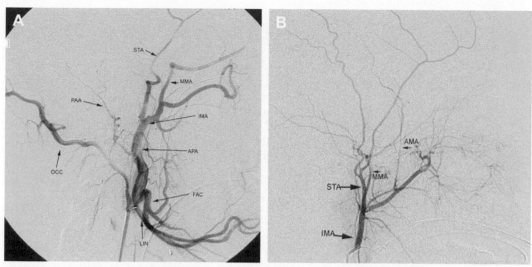

Fig. 9. Lateral ECA arteriogram demonstrates the typical branching pattern of the ECA (*A, B*). (PAA, posterior auricular; MMA, middle meningeal; AMA, accessory meningeal).

the vertebral artery that provides the larger percentage of posterior fossa vascular supply. Approximately 50% of the time, the left vertebral artery is dominant, 25% it is the right vertebral artery, with no distinction in the remainder.[13,16–18]

As the vertebral arteries proceed through the dura at the level of the foramen magnum they join to form a common basilar artery. The posterior inferior cerebellar artery (PICA) is a large, variable branch of the vertebral artery usually arising proximal to the origin of the basilar artery; however, it can arise as single or multiple branches, arise from the proximal basilar artery, or may represent the terminal branch of the vertebral artery in cases where there is no communication with the basilar artery. The PICA enjoys a balanced circulation with branches of the anterior inferior cerebellar artery (AICA) and not uncommonly an AICA-PICA variant exists when the AICA supplies the distal PICA territory and the PICA is absent or vice versa[13,19,20] The posterior spinal artery is also often a proximal branch of the intracranial

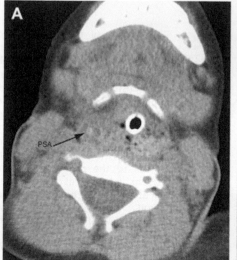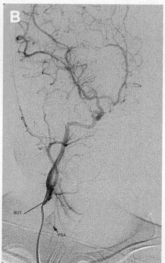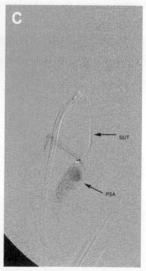

Fig.10. (*A*) Five-year-old child 9 days post tonsillectomy with massive oral bleeding; axial contrast CT demonstrates a contrast collection (*arrow*) in the inferior aspect of the operative bed. (*B*) Oblique AP right CCA arteriogram reveals a focal blush arising from the superior thyroid (SUT) artery. (*C*) Microcatheterization of the SUT reveals the pseudoaneurysm (PSA) which was embolized with *n* butyl cyanoacrylate (NBCA).

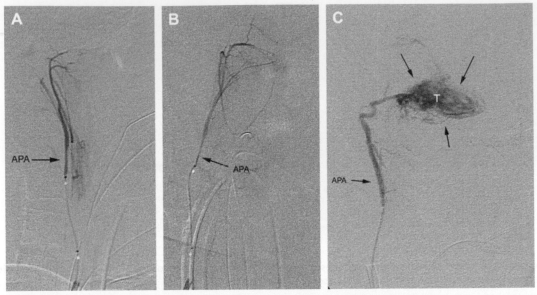

Fig. 11. (*A, B*) Lateral and AP selective arteriograms of the normal APA. (*C*) Hypertrophy of the normal APA supplying this hypervascular juvenile nasal angiofibroma invading the skull base.

vertebral artery and may occasionally arise from the PICA, whereas the anterior spinal artery arises from the distal end of the vertebral artery and descends anterior to the medulla oblongata joining the contralateral anterior spinal artery and descending as a single vessel with segmental perforators to supply the anterior spinal cord (**Fig. 7**A). Posterior meningeal branches (dural) arise from the cervical vertebral artery, and sometimes from the PICA, to supply bone and dura of the posterior fossa, and potential dural vascular supply to dural arteriovenous malformations (**Fig. 7**B).[13]

COMMON CAROTID ARTERIES

After arising from the aortic arch, the common carotid arteries proceed cephalad within the fibrous carotid sheath in the neck along with the internal jugular vein, the vagus nerve, and the ansa cervicalis. The cervical portion of the common carotid artery (CCA) has no normal branches before the carotid bifurcation, with rare exceptions.[21] The terminal portion of the CCA dilates mildly, and is referred to as the carotid bulb, and then bifurcates into the internal

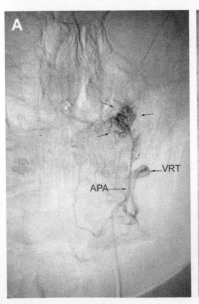

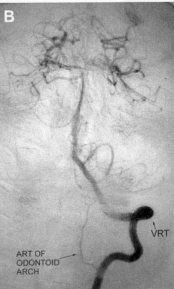

Fig. 12. Artery of the odontoid arch. (*A*) Selective APA injection before embolization of skull base giant cell tumor (arrows) demonstrates a midline vessel filling the vertebral from the APA. (*B*) Note the vessel filling on the selective vertebral artery injection. Safe embolization requires the catheter position distal to the collateral branch. (*From* Johnson et al. Vascular anatomy of the head, neck, and skull base. In Hurst RW, Rosenwasser RH, editors. Interventional neuroradiology. New York: Taylor and Frances; 2007; with permission.)

and external carotid arteries between the levels of the thyroid cartilage and the greater horn of the hyoid bone (C1-C2 to C6-C7) (**Fig. 8**).[2,22,23] Surgically, the facial vein often serves as a landmark for localization of the carotid bifurcation. In approximately 80% of patients, the bifurcation is located between the C3 and C5 levels,[23,24] with the anatomic location more important for surgical access than for endovascular approaches.

EXTERNAL CAROTID ARTERIES

The ECA arises from the CCA at the bulb and supplies the face, orbit, scalp, and dura. There are multiple potential anastomotic channels to the intracranial internal carotid and extracranial vertebral, as well as to branches of the proximal subclavian arteries.[5,24] External carotid branches are variable in size and distribution and there is a rich anastomotic network between ipsilateral branches and between contralateral branches

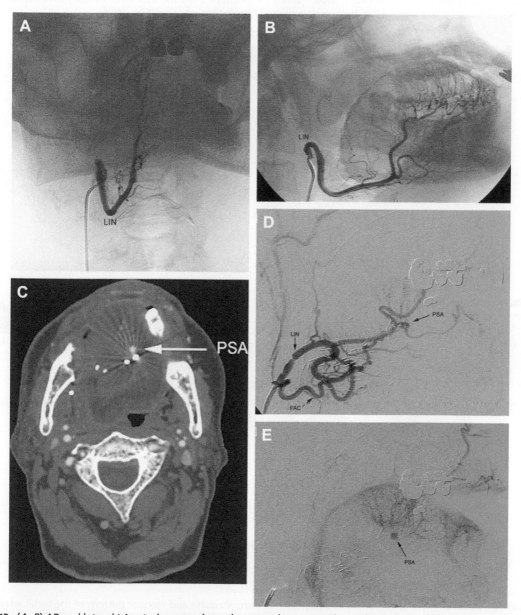

Fig. 13. (*A*, *B*) AP and lateral LA arteriograms show the normal course and vascular pattern of the tongue. (*B*) Axial CTA in a patient with oral cancer and intermittent oral bleeding reveals a contrast collection adjacent to the brachytherapy seeds, consistent with pseudoaneurysm (PSA) (*C*). Early (*D*) and late (*E*) phase lingual arteriography reveal the PSA within the oral tongue. Note the normal variant common lingual/facial trunk (*D*).

within the face. Occasionally, several ECA branches may arise separately from the common carotid trunk, and rarely the external carotid may arise directly from the aortic arch, separate from the internal carotid artery (ICA).[25–27] The ECA courses from its origin at the common carotid bifurcation along the lateral pharyngeal wall and passes beneath the posterior belly of the digastric and stylohyoid muscles to pierce the carotid fascia. The deep lobe of the parotid gland separates the ECA from the ICA.[1,5,6]

Two organizational schemes have been proposed to categorize the ECA branches either craniocaudally or anteriorly/posteriorly to predict the vascular source of bleeding or of neovascularity on the basis of cross-sectional imaging. The first divides the external carotid branches into 3 craniocaudal segments: (1) lower to cervical; (2) middle to mandibular angle; and (3) upper to parotid. The second scheme divides the ECA branches into an anterior group (superior thyroid, lingual, and facial arteries), and a posterior group (ascending pharyngeal, occipital, and posterior auricular arteries). The ECA terminal branches are the internal maxillary and superficial temporal arteries (**Fig. 9**).[24]

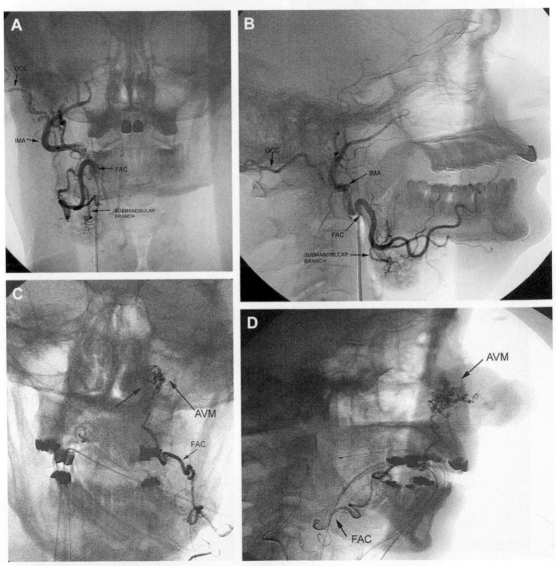

Fig. 14. (*A, B*) AP and lateral ECA arteriograms show the normal course and vascular pattern of the facial artery in relation to adjacent ECA branches. Note the prominent submandibular branch and the pattern of submandibular gland vascularity. (*C, D*) AP and lateral unsubtracted selective FAC arteriograms illustrate the FAC distal branches that normally supply the nose and nasal mucosa. These vessels are enlarged in this patient with a large nasal arteriovenous malformation (AVM).

Superior Thyroid Artery

The superior thyroid artery (SUT) is usually the most proximal branch of the ECA, although it may arise from the carotid bifurcation or directly from the CCA on occasion.[24–28] The SUT courses inferiorly alongside the thyroid gland to provide supply to the superior pole of thyroid gland and the larynx and can be readily identified by the prominent thyroid blush after arterial contrast injection (see **Fig. 4**D). Extensive collaterals exist between the contralateral superior thyroid artery and the inferior thyroid artery originating from the thyrocervical trunk (branch of subclavian artery). Rare injury to the SUT may occur following laryngeal or tonsilar surgery with resultant bleeding or pseudoaneurysm formation (**Fig. 10**).

Ascending Pharyngeal Artery

The ascending pharyngeal artery (APA) is the most proximal posterior ECA branch and ascends from its origin from the ECA to parallel the course of the internal carotid artery, coursing just deep to the pharyngeal mucosal space.[5] The APA can occasionally be mistaken for the ICA on ultrasound particularly in the setting of internal carotid artery occlusion, (a source of false-positive ultrasound screening).[29] The APA divides into an anterior division, supplying the pharynx and eustachian tube, and a posterior division supplying the tympanic

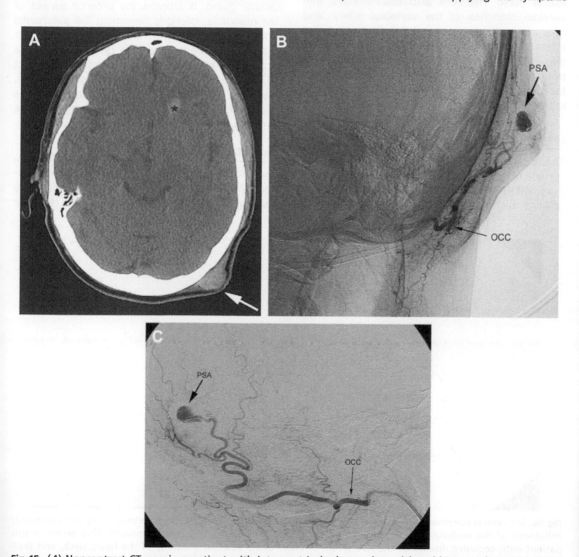

Fig. 15. (A) Noncontrast CT scan in a patient with intraventricular hemorrhage (*) and history of recent surgical excision of a scalp mass had a residual painful and pulsatile subcutaneous mass (arrow). (B, C) Selective oblique and lateral occipital artery arteriography demonstrates a pseudoaneurysm (PSA) of the distal OCC treated with NBCA.

cavity and pre-vertebral musculature (**Fig. 11**A, B). The neuromeningeal branch is small, but clinically important, supplying the dura and the lower cranial nerves. The APA provides significant contribution to the vascular supply to tumors of the jugular foramen, such as glomus jugulare tumors, and tumors invading the skull base, such as aggressive juvenile angiofibromas (**Fig. 11**C). From its location just below the skull base, the APA provides extensive anastomoses to middle meningeal and accessory meningeal branches of the ECA, and to the ICA via the inferior tympanic artery, which anastomoses with the caroticotympanic artery from the petrous ICA.[24,30] There are variable anastomoses between the APA, the vidian artery, and the inferolateral trunk. The APA also anastomoses with cervical branches of the vertebral artery, and may provide a direct connection to the vertebral artery via the artery of the odontoid arch (**Fig. 12**).[2] Angiographic recognition of these potential intracranial collaterals is critically important before endovascular embolization of lesions in the APA territory.[24,30]

Lingual Artery

The lingual artery (LIN) arises from the anterior surface of the ECA, and may arise from a common trunk with the facial artery (FAC). The LIN loops upward and courses anteriorly along the hyoid and deep into the hypoglossal muscle to supply the ipsilateral tongue, sublingual gland, the pharynx, and hyoid musculature.[1,2,24] A characteristic U-shape and the ramifications of the branches within the tongue musculature distinguish this vessel angiographically (**Fig. 13**A, B) Injury to the LIN may result in erosion or laceration with pseudoaneurysm formation and massive bleeding (**Fig. 13**C–E).

Facial Artery

The FAC is the third anteriorly oriented ECA branch and ascends along the superior constrictor muscle, passing deep into the stylohyoid and digastric muscles and coursing over the submandibular gland. It crosses the anterior aspect of the mandible, inferiorly becoming the submental artery supplying the mouth and submandibular gland. The superior branches of the FAC course obliquely superiorly from the inferolateral aspect of the face to provide supply to the lips, palate, pharynx, and nasal cavity floor, terminating as the angular artery near the medial canthus of the eye (**Fig. 14**).[1,2,24]

Occipital Artery

The occipital artery (OCC) is the next distal posterior branch arising opposite the facial artery passing beneath the posterior belly of the digastric

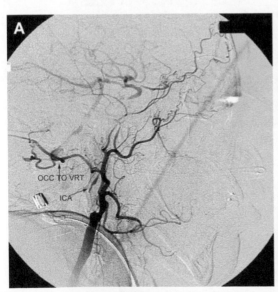
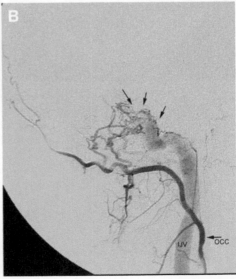

Fig. 16. (*A*) Lateral common carotid injection demonstrates prompt filling of the vertebral artery from muscular collaterals of the occipital artery. The anterior circulation fills via the posterior communicating artery in this patient with occlusive disease of the ICA. (*From* Johnson et al. Vascular anatomy of the head, neck, and skull base. In Hurst RW, Rosenwasser RH, editors. Interventional neuroradiology. New York: Taylor and Frances; 2007; with permission.) (*B*) Selective occipital arteriography demonstrates enlarged dural branches of the OCC with fistulization (arrows) to the transverse sinus and shunting into the sinus and jugular vein (IJV) in this patient with dural AVM and tinnitus.

and sternocleidomastoid muscles and giving rise to muscular penetrating branches. The occipital artery courses within the subcutaneous tissues of the posterior scalp supplying the posterior skin, muscles, and meninges of the posterior fossa.[1,2,24,31] The subcutaneous course of the OCC, and that of the superficial temporal artery (see later discussion) make both arteries subject to direct injury and pseudoaneurysms may develop, commonly presenting as pulsatile "lumps" on the forehead or scalp following remote, often minor trauma (**Fig. 15**). Prominent muscular collaterals exist between the occipital arteries and the vertebral arteries and may represent a significant source of collateral flow in the setting of vertebral artery stenosis or occlusion. Meningeal (dural) branches of the occipital artery pass intracranially via the hypoglossal and mastoid canals and the jugular foramen, and often become enlarged in the setting of dural arteriovenous malformation (**Fig. 16**).

Posterior Auricular Artery

The posterior auricular artery (PAA) arises from the posterior aspect of the ECA just above the level of the OCC and may occasionally arise from a common trunk or as a branch of the OCC.[1,2,24] The PAA stylomastoid branch traverses the stylomastoid foramen and provides branches to the chorda tympani within the tympanic cavity, and to the mastoid and semicircular canals and anastomoses with petrosal branches of the middle meningeal artery. The auricular branch supplies the scalp, the pinna, and the external auditory canal. A normal blush of the pinna can be seen at angiography of the PAA (**Fig. 17**).

Superficial Temporal Artery

The ECA terminates within the parotid gland at its bifurcation into the superficial temporal artery (STA) and the internal maxillary artery (IMA). The STA courses over the zygomatic arch dividing

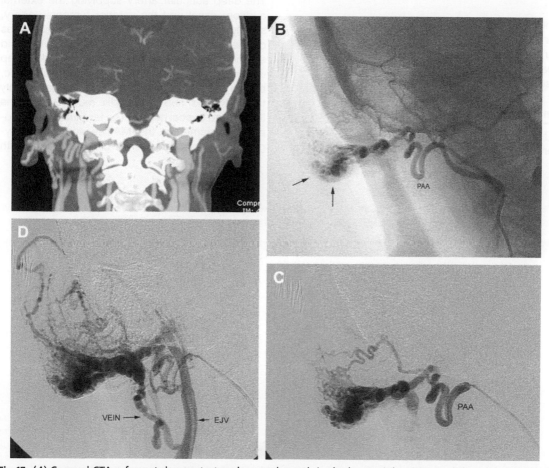

Fig. 17. (*A*) Coronal CTA reformat demonstrates abnormal vessels in the lower right pinna and prominent cervical veins. (*B*) Oblique unsubtracted posterior auricular angiogram shows the AVM of the inferior pinna. Early (*C*) and late (*D*) microcatheter angiograms reveal the architecture of the AVM and the shunting into the EJV.

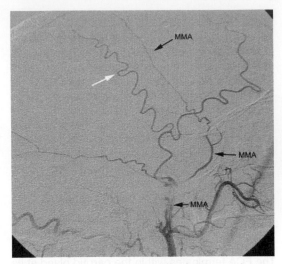

Fig. 18. Lateral view from a distal ECA angiogram demonstrates the course of the MMA. Note the straight dural MMA branch (*black arrow*) compared with the undulating course of the scalp branches of the STA (*white arrow*).

into frontal and parietal branches that supply the anterior two thirds of the scalp, the underlying cranium and musculature, and portions of the parotid gland, pinna, and temporomandibular joint (see **Fig. 9**).[1,2,24]

Internal Maxillary Artery

The IMA courses deep to the neck of the mandible, enters the temporal fossa passing horizontally between the heads of the medial and lateral pterygoid muscles, through the pterygomaxillary fissure, and into the pterygopalatine fossa.[1,2,5,6,24] The IMA is divided into 3 segments defined by the position of the artery relative to the pterygoid muscle. The proximal segment can rise to the inferior alveolar artery and extends along with the mandibular nerve to the mandibular foramen. The middle meningeal artery (MMA) and accessory meningeal artery (AMA) pass through the foramen spinosum and ovale respectively (see **Fig. 9**B). As the MMA ascends superiorly from the IMA, it forms a curve that parallels the sella after it exits the foramen spinosum. Occasionally, the MMA may give rise to or arise from the ophthalmic artery (OPH).[32]

Meningeal branches can be differentiated from scalp branches angiographically by their characteristic straight, rather than tortuous, course. Remembering that "you can wrinkle your forehead, but you cannot wrinkle your dura" is a helpful key to differentiating these branches (**Fig. 18**).[2] The deep auricular artery supplying the external auditory canal and the anterior tympanic artery, supplying the tympanic membrane are branches of the first segment of the IMA. The pterygoid segment (middle) is located in the high, deep masticator space and gives rise to masseteric, buccal, and deep temporal arteries that supply the pterygoid and temporalis muscles and the lingual and buccal nerves. The terminal or sphenopalatine segment of the IMA lies within the pterygopalatine fossa and sends branches along with

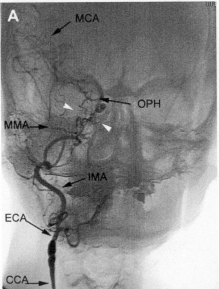

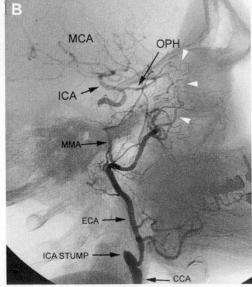

Fig. 19. AP (*A*) and lateral (*B*) common carotid angiograms in a patient with asymptomatic ICA occlusion demonstrates robust collateralization from ethmoidal branches of the distal IMA to ethmoidal branches of the OPH and retrograde OPH flow to reconstitute the intracranial ICA and middle cerebral artery (MCA) branches.

each nerve to the pterygopalatine ganglion. The IMA terminates in multiple branches to the nasal cavity supplying both nasal wall and septum, the posterior superior alveolar artery supplying the palate and posterior maxilla and the infraorbital artery that traverses the infraorbital fissure along the orbital floor to perfuse the inferior orbital contents. Ethmoidal branches of the distal IMA represent an important source of collateral flow in the setting of carotid occlusive disease (see later discussion) (**Fig. 19**).[30]

External Carotid Anastomotic Network

The importance of ECA to ICA collaterals and potential anastomotic pathways cannot be over-emphasized in the setting of disease and neurointervention.[1,2,5,24,33] Such interconnections are dynamic, may not be visible on the baseline control arteriogram, and may change in appearance and flow during the intervention. These collateral channels often become most dangerous near the end of the procedure. For example, the IMA has numerous extensive anastomoses with

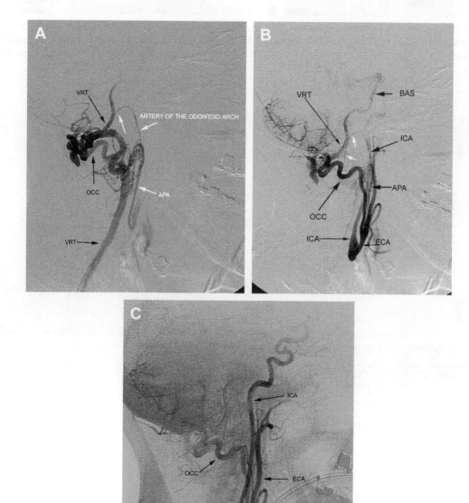

Fig. 20. Sequential lateral early (*A*), late arterial (*B*), and venous phase (*C*) vertebral arteriography in a patient with remote surgical ligation of the CCA demonstrates reconstitution of the ECA via the artery of the odontoid arch to the APA and from muscular collaterals from the vertebral artery to the occipital artery. The flow is retrograde from these branches then the CCA bifurcation fills and the flow into the internal carotid is antegrade.

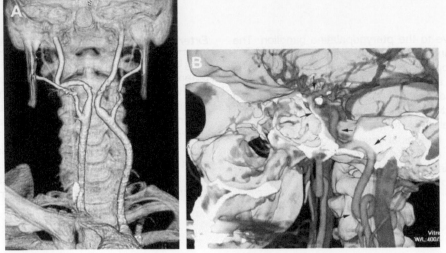

Fig. 21. (*A*) Three-dimensional Vitrea reformat demonstrates the CCA arising from the aortic arch and a variant medial course of the ICAs referred to as "kissing carotids." (*B*) Oblique cutaway three-dimensional Vitrea reformat demonstrates a cervical ICA loop and the course of the intracranial ICA (*arrows*) in relation to the bony landmarks.

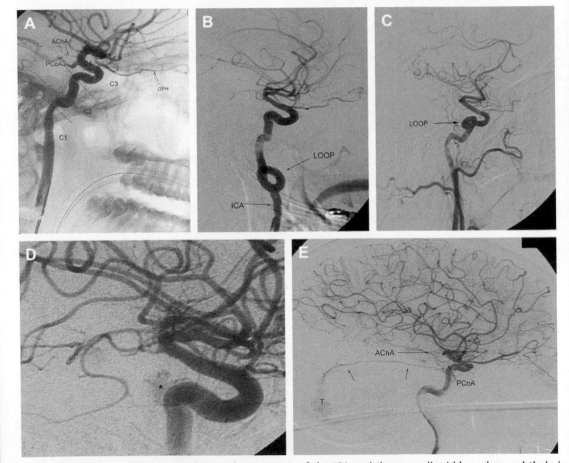

Fig. 22. (*A*) Lateral ICA arteriogram depicts the segments of the ICA and the supraclinoid branches, ophthalmic (OPH), posterior communicating (PCoA) and anterior choroidal (AChA). (*B*) An ICA loop is a normal variant. (*C*) This ICA loop at the petrous cavernous junction is an unusual variant. (*D*) The normal "pituitary blush" (*) is identified on this lateral ICA angiogram. (*E*) The tentorial artery (arrows) is markedly enlarged and supplies a dural AVM draining into the transverse sinus (T).

other ECA branches in the face, both ipsilateral and contralateral.

With ECA to ICA anastomoses, flow may proceed in either direction, dependent on the location and nature of the diseased vasculature, and how long the flow compromise has been present. Distal ethmoidal branches of the IMA collateralize with distal ethmoidal branches of the OPH, thus providing a supply route to the supraclinoid ICA with reversal of flow through the OPH (see **Fig. 19**). The vidian artery collateralizes with the petrous ICA and the artery of the foramen rotundum and the inferolateral trunk anastomose with the cavernous ICA.[5,24,30] These

ECA-ICA anastomoses vary among patients and may represent clinically significant collateral pathways in the setting of occlusive vascular disease. In extreme cases, ECA-ICA collaterals can reconstitute flow to the ICA via vertebral-to-ECA collaterals resulting in retrograde filling of major ECA branches and reconstitution of the ICA (**Fig. 20**).[5,24,30]

Internal Carotid Artery

Nomenclature varies, but the 4-part division of the ICA, designated as C1-C4 and described in the radiology and surgical literature, is useful (**Fig. 21**).[2,34,35] The cervical segment (C1) begins

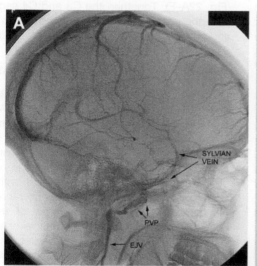

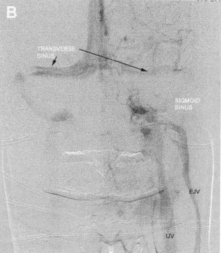

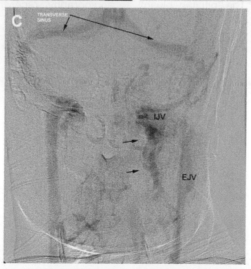

Fig. 23. (A) Lateral LCCA angiogram in venous phase demonstrates normal variation in venous drainage from the sylvian (greater middle cerebral) vein to the PVP and to the EJV. Venous phase angiogram in patient with subjective tinnitus (B) neutral position and (C) head turned to the left with filming AP for comparison. In neutral (B), note filling of the IJV and EJV on the left. With head turned (C), the tinnitus increased and there is enlargement and preferential filling of the EJV and posterior cervical vein (arrows) and more pronounced filling of the contralateral IJV.

proximally at the origin of the ICA with the CCA and extends cephalad to the external orifice of the carotid canal. C1 does not normally have branches. The ICA enters the skull base at the carotid canal and ascends anterior to the jugular bulb and posterior to the eustachian tube as the petrous (C2) segment.[1,5,6,36] After traversing the carotid canal, the ICA courses anteromedial to the middle ear (tympanic cavity), and over the foramen lacerum to enter the dura of the cavernous sinus (see **Fig. 21**). The C2 (petrous) segment gives rise to the caroticotympanic artery (supplying the middle and inner ear), the vidian artery, a.k.a. the artery of the pterygoid canal, which goes through the foramen lacerum; and the artery of the foramen rotundum, along with variable periosteal branches.[35–37] The C3 or cavernous segment begins with its entry into the cavernous sinus dura and ends where the ICA pierces the dural roof of the cavernous sinus.[37–39] C3 gives rise to 3 branches or trunks. The posterior trunk, or the meningohypophyseal trunk, also has 3 branches: (1) the tentorial artery (of Bernasconi and Casinari) supplying the tentorium; (2) the inferior hypophyseal artery supplying the posterior pituitary capsule; and (3) the dorsal meningeal artery supplying the abducens nerve and the clivus (**Fig. 22**A).[37–40] The lateral trunk, or inferior cavernous sinus artery, gives supply to the inferolateral cavernous sinus wall and region of the foramen ovale and spinosum. The medial trunk, or McConnell capsular artery (present in only 28% of the population), supplies the anterior and inferior pituitary capsule.[36–39] The "pituitary blush"

is commonly identified on lateral ICA arteriograms (**Fig. 22**D). These C3 branches provide potential anastomoses with ECA in the setting of occlusive disease and provide neovascular supply to tumors of the central skull base.[2,36–39]

The supraclinoid segment (C4) begins where the ICA exits the dural ring and enters the subarachnoid space, and it ends at the internal carotid bifurcation into anterior and middle cerebral artery branches.[3,8,9,34,35,37–39] C4 courses medial to the anterior clinoid process and below the optic nerve. Branches include the OPH, the superior hypophyseal artery, the posterior communicating artery (or the variant fetal origin of the posterior cerebral artery), and the anterior choroidal artery (**Fig. 22**A–E). Together, the C3 and C4 segments form the characteristic "S" shape seen on lateral and oblique angiographic views of the skull base.

VEINS OF THE HEAD, NECK, AND SKULL BASE

Facial venous drainage is largely superficial with drainage into the external jugular vein (EJV). The supraorbital and supratrochlear veins of the face join to become the angular vein, which subsequently becomes the facial vein at the angle of the mandible.[1,5,6] The pterygopalatine venous plexus (PVP) is located around and within the lateral pterygoid muscle and may be recognized on contrast CT as a focal area of irregular enhancement adjacent to the muscle or as flow voids surrounding the pterygoid musculature on MRI. The PVP is frequently identified on cerebral angiography receiving flow from the greater

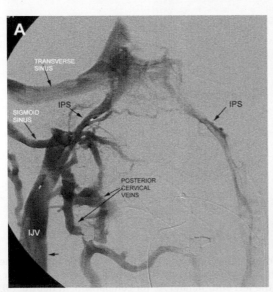
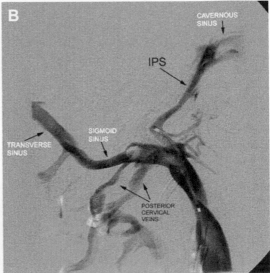

Fig. 24. AP (*A*) and lateral (*B*) views of and internal jugular venogram with microcatheters in place before IPS sampling for pituitary Cushings demonstrates normal venous anatomy. Note the cavernous sinus filling and the contralateral IPS filling via the cavernous sinus and clival venous plexus.

middle cerebral (sylvian) vein (a normal variant) **(Fig. 23)**. The PVP drains into a pair of maxillary veins, which lie deep to the neck of the mandible and join with the temporalis vein, which drains the temporal region of the face and scalp, to form the retromandibular vein. The inferior ophthalmic vein courses with the infraorbital artery and normally drains into the cavernous sinus intracranially and into the PVP extracranially. The facial veins may occasionally drain superiorly into the ophthalmic veins and subsequently into the cavernous sinus as a normal variation in the absence of arteriovenous malformation or shunting.[41] The retromandibular vein passes through the parotid gland and divides into anterior and posterior branches that drain into the internal and external jugular veins (IJV and EJV), respectively. The deep facial vein represents the anastomosis between the PVP and the facial vein. The anterior jugular veins lie in the submental region extending inferiorly to the suprasternal notch, where they drain into the EJV deep to the sternocleidomastoid muscle. The posterior auricular vein also drains into the EJV. The EJV empties into the subclavian vein near the midpoint of the clavicle. The IJV originates from the jugular bulb receiving blood from the sigmoid sinus and its first extracranial tributary, the inferior petrosal sinus (IPS) **(Fig. 24)**.[41,42] The IJV courses inferiorly, posterior to the ICA directly adjacent to the arch of C1, where it joins the subclavian vein to become the brachiocephalic vein. The left brachiocephalic vein joins the right just to the right of the second costal cartilage to become the superior vena cava.

SUMMARY

Understanding the normal and variant anatomy of the head, neck, and skull base is critical to the development of accurate diagnosis, and for the development of safe and effective treatment strategies for vascular and nonvascular lesions. Localization, anticipation of vascular supply, and knowledge of potential collaterals and dangerous anastomoses are important precursors to patient management.

REFERENCES

1. Johnson MH. Head and neck vascular anatomy. Neuroimaging Clin N Am 1998;8:119–41.
2. Johnson MH, Thorisson HM, DiLuna ML. Vascular anatomy of the head, neck, and skull base. In: Hurst RW, Rosenwasser RH, editors. Interventional neuroradiology. New York: Taylor and Frances Group, LLC; 2007.
3. Langman J. Medical embryology. 3rd edition. Baltimore (MD): William & Wilkins; 1975.
4. Haughton VM, Rosenbaum AE. The normal and anomalous aortic arch and brachiocephalic vessels. In: Newton TH, Potts GN, editors. Radiology of the skull and brain: angiography, vol. 2. Great Neck (NY): Mosby; 1974. p. 1145–63.
5. Gray S. Gray's anatomy. 1st edition. New York: Vintage Books; 1994.
6. Last RJ, McMinn RMH. Last's anatomy, regional and applied. 9th edition. Edinburgh: New York: Churchill Livingstone; 1994.
7. Faggioli GL, Ferri M, Freyrie A, et al. Aortic arch anomalies are associated with increased risk of neurologic events in carotid stent procedures. Eur J Vasc Endovasc Surg 2007;33:436–41.
8. De Garis C, Black I, Riemenschneider E. Patterns of the aortic arch in American white and Negro stocks, with comparative notes on certain other mammals. J Anat 1933;67:599–619.
9. Layton KF, Kallmes DF, Cloft HJ, et al. Bovine aortic arch variant in humans: clarification of a common misnomer. AJNR Am J Neuroradiol 2006;27:1541–2.
10. Lemke AJ, Benndorf G, Liebig T, et al. Anomalous origin of the right vertebral artery: review of the literature and case report of right vertebral artery origin distal to the left subclavian artery. AJNR Am J Neuroradiol 1999;20:1318–21.
11. Caus T, Gaubert JY, Monties JR, et al. Right-sided aortic arch: surgical treatment of an aneurysm arising from a Kommerell's diverticulum and extending to the descending thoracic aorta with an aberrant left subclavian artery. Cardiovasc Surg 1994; 2(1):110–3.
12. Cina CS, Arena GO, Bruin G, et al. Kommerell's diverticulum and aneurysmal right-sided aortic arch: a case report and review of the literature. J Vasc Surg 2000;32(6):1208–14.
13. Newton TH, Mani RL. The vertebral artery. In: Newton TH, Potts DG, editors. Angiography. St. Louis (MO): Mosby; 1974. p. 1659–709.
14. Kashimada A, Machida K, Honda N, et al. Measurement of cerebral blood flow with two-dimensional cine phase-contrast mR imaging: evaluation of normal subjects and patients with vertigo. Radiat Med 1995;13:95–102.
15. Paksoy Y, Vatansev H, Seker M, et al. Congenital morphological abnormalities of the distal vertebral arteries (CMADVA) and their relationship with vertigo and dizziness. Med Sci Monit 2004;10: CR316–23.
16. Mitchell J. Differences between left and right suboccipital and intracranial vertebral artery dimensions: an influence on blood flow to the hindbrain? Physiother Res Int 2004;9:85–95.
17. Seidel E, Eicke BM, Tettenborn B, et al. Reference values for vertebral artery flow volume by duplex

sonography in young and elderly adults. Stroke 1999;30:2692–6.

18. Smith AS, Bellon JR. Parallel and spiral flow patterns of vertebral artery contributions to the basilar artery. AJNR Am J Neuroradiol 1995;16:1587–91.

19. Johnson MH, Christman CW. Posterior circulation infarction: anatomy, pathophysiology, and clinical correlation. Semin Ultrasound CT MR 1995;16:237.

20. Lister JR, Rhoton AL Jr, Matsushima T, et al. Microsurgical anatomy of the posterior inferior cerebellar artery. Neurosurgery 1982;10:170–99, 23.

21. Matsumoto M, Okuda H, Ishidoh E, et al. An anomalous case of the common carotid artery giving off several branches and high division of the internal carotid artery. Okajimas Folia Anat Jpn 1986;63:37–43.

22. Lo A, Oehley M, Bartlett A, et al. Anatomical variations of the common carotid artery bifurcation. ANZ J Surg 2006;76:970–2.

23. Thomas JB, Antiga L, Che SL, et al. Variation in the carotid bifurcation geometry of young versus older adults: implications for geometric risk of atherosclerosis. Stroke 2005;36:2450–6.

24. Djindian R, Merland J. Normal superselective arteriography of the external carotid artery. In: Djindian R, Merland J, editors. Superselective arteriography of the external carotid artery. New York: Springer-Verlag; 1978. p. 1–46.

25. Cakirer S, Karaarslan E. Aortic arch origin of the left external carotid artery. AJNR Am J Neuroradiol 2003;24:1492 [author reply 1492].

26. Morimoto T, Nitta K, Kazekawa K, et al. The anomaly of a non-bifurcating cervical carotid artery. Case report. J Neurosurg 1990;72:130–2.

27. Ooigawa H, Nawashiro H, Fukui S, et al. Non-bifurcating cervical carotid artery. J Clin Neurosci 2006;13:944–7.

28. Toni R, Della Casa C, Castorina S, et al. A meta-analysis of superior thyroid artery variations in different human groups and their clinical implications. Ann Anat 2004;186:255–62.

29. Wei CJ, Chang FC, Chiou SY, et al. Aberrant ascending pharyngeal artery mimicking a partially occluded internal carotid artery. J Neuroimaging 2004;14:67–70.

30. Mishkin M, Schreiber M. Collateral circulation. In: Newton T, Potts D, editors. Radiology of the skull and brain, vol. 2. St. Louis (MO): Mosby; 1977. p. 2344–74.

31. Alvernia JE, Fraser K, Lanzino G. The occipital artery: a microanatomical study. Neurosurgery 2006;58:ONS114–22.

32. Kawai K, Yoshinaga K, Koizumi M, et al. A middle meningeal artery which arises from the internal carotid artery in which the first branchial artery participates. Ann Anat 2006;188:33–8.

33. Johnson MH, Chiang VL, Ross DA. Interventional neuroradiology adjuncts and alternatives in patients with head and neck vascular lesions. Neurosurg Clin N Am 2005;16:547–60.

34. Day AL. Aneurysms of the ophthalmic segment. A clinical and anatomical analysis. J Neurosurg 1990;72:677–91.

35. Rhoton A. Rhoton's cranial anatomy and surgical approaches. Schaumburg (IL): Lippincott Williams & Wilkins; 2003.

36. Lasjuanias P, Berenstein A. The internal carotid artery (ICA). In: Lasjuanias P, Berenstein A, editors. Surgical neuroimaging: functional vascular anatomy of brain, spinal cord and spine. 3rd edition. Berlin: Springer-Verlag; 1990.

37. Tubbs RS, Hansasuta A, Loukas M, et al. Branches of the petrous and cavernous segments of the internal carotid artery. Clin Anat 2007;20:596–601.

38. Harris F, Rhoton AL Jr. Microsurgical anatomy of the cavernous sinus. Surg Forum 1975;26:462–3.

39. Harris FS, Rhoton AL. Anatomy of the cavernous sinus. A microsurgical study. J Neurosurg 1976;45:169–80.

40. Worthington C, Olivier A, Melanson D. Internal carotid artery agenesis: correlation by conventional and digital subtraction angiography, and by computed tomography. Surg Neurol 1984;22:295–300.

41. Hacker H. Normal supratentorial veins and dural sinuses. In: Newton TH, Potts DG, editors. Radiology of the skull and brain. Great Neck (NY): Mosby; 1974. p. 1851.

42. Huang Y, Wolf B. Veins of the posterior fossa. In: Newton TH, Potts DG, editors. Radiology of the skull and brain, vol. 2. Great Neck (NY): Mosby; 1974. p. 2155.

The Vascular Anatomy of the Vertebro-Spinal Axis

Tibor Becske, MD[a,b,c], Peter Kim Nelson, MD[a,b,c],*

KEYWORDS

- Spinal cord • Anterior spinal artery
- Posterior spinal artery • Spinal vasculature

The vascular supply of the spinal axis is systematically determined during the first few weeks of development as a consequence of the somatotopic organization of the spine.[1] During this embryologic interval, 31 somites are formed, each receiving one individual pair of segmental arteries from the dorsal aorta. These paired segmental arteries ultimately support a functionally distinct vascular compartment comprising each developing metamere. The thoracolumbar spinal vasculature (**Fig. 1**) retains the classically paired segmental arrangement into adulthood, with minor changes in appearance attributed to differences in the longitudinal growth of the spinal cord and vertebral column, respectively, during skeletal maturation. This disparity in comparative length accounts for the increasing obliquity of the nerve roots and, correspondingly, the radicular arteries and veins in relation to their named intercostal or segmental levels.

By comparison, considerable modification of the segmental disposition occurs throughout the cervical spine. The development of serially consecutive intersegmental anastomoses establishes three dominant craniocaudal vascular channels (from anterior to posterior): the anterior cervical artery, the vertebral artery, and the deep cervical artery, each of which may independently and variably participate in the vascularization of vertebrae, paraspinal musculature, and cervical spinal cord (**Fig. 2**). With respect to the developing sacrum, paired lateral sacral arteries (**Fig. 3**) arise from the internal iliac arteries to supply the sacral nerve roots, vertebrae, and paraspinal musculature. Medially, the distal dorsal aorta regresses to become the middle sacral artery, which anastomoses laterally with corresponding branches of the lateral sacral arteries at the sacral neuroforamina.

VASCULAR SUPPLY TO THE SPINE, SPINAL DURA, AND PARASPINAL MUSCULATURE

From an angiographic standpoint, the arterial supply to the bony spine, spinal canal, and paravertebral muscles may be divided into four vascular territories at each vertebral level:[2–4] (1) The main intercostal or lumbar segmental arteries provide fine branches to the anterolateral aspect of the vertebral body before giving off the dorsal spinal trunk. (2) The ventral division of the dorsal spinal artery supplies the structures of the spinal canal, including the bony elements, epidural space, dura, and contents of the thecal sac. Anteriorly, an arterial arcade situated beneath the posterior longitudinal ligament vascularizes the posterior surface of the vertebral body. Posteriorly, branches run in the posterior epidural space to supply the anterior aspect of the lamina and a portion of the spinous process. (3) The dorsal division of the dorsal spinal artery ultimately passes posteriorly beneath the ipsilateral transverse process and along the outer surface of the lamina, forming an arterial plexus close to the

[a] Department of Neurology, New York University, Langone Medical Center, 560 First Avenue Room HE208, New York, NY 10016, USA
[b] Department of Neurosurgery, New York University, Langone Medical Center, 560 First Avenue Room HE208, New York, NY 10016, USA
[c] Department of Radiology, New York University, Langone Medical Center, 560 First Avenue Room HE208, New York, NY 10016, USA
* Corresponding author. Department of Neurology, New York University, Langone Medical Center, 560 First Avenue Room HE208, New York, NY 10016.
E-mail address: Peter.Nelson@nyumc.org (P.K. Nelson).

Neurosurg Clin N Am 20 (2009) 259–264
doi:10.1016/j.nec.2009.03.002
1042-3680/09/$ – see front matter © 2009 Elsevier Inc. All rights reserved.

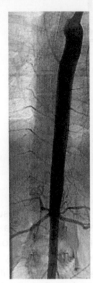

Fig. 1. Aortogram, frontal projection. Paired segmental arrangement of thoracolumbar spinal vessels.

spinous process and providing middle and lateral muscular branches to the dorsal muscular groups. (4) Each thoracic and lumbar segmental artery also supplies lateral muscular branches, which in the thoracic region are reflected beneath each rib as the continuation of the intercostal arteries.

When viewed from the perspective of the spinal column, specific intraspinal and extraspinal anastomoses may be described between adjacent segmental vessels. These anastomotic connections occur between successive vertebral levels along a longitudinal axis and through transverse anastomoses across the midline. Within the spinal canal, transverse anastomoses are present dorsal and ventral to the dural sheath, forming an extra-dural ring, several branches of which supply the adjacent bony and dural structures. Branch arteries entering the epidural space anteriorly characteristically divide into a hexagonal branching pattern recognizable angiographically as the retrocorporeal collateral arcade (**Fig. 4**). The ascending limb of this arterial network vascularizes the posterior aspect of its segmentally named vertebral body and anastomoses with its contralateral complement and descending epidural branches from the segmental arteries of the level above, establishing transverse and longitudinal collateral interconnections within the anterior epidural space.

Longitudinal anastomoses additionally exist between the extraspinal branches of consecutive segmental arteries (**Fig. 5**). Ventrally, they typically are divided into anterior, anterolateral, and pretransverse groups, the latter participating in the supply of the sympathetic nervous system. Dorsally, longitudinal anastomoses exist between successive dorsal muscular branches adjacent to the spinous processes. If coupled to regression of primary thoracic and lumbar segmental arteries, compensatory enlargement of these longitudinal collaterals may give rise to anatomic variations in intercostal and spinal supply (**Fig. 6**). As indicated in the discussion of the cervical spinal vasculature, the development of dominant longitudinal extraspinal anastomoses throughout the cervical levels establishes the ascending cervical, vertebral, and deep cervical arteries on which the vascularization of the cervical spine depends.

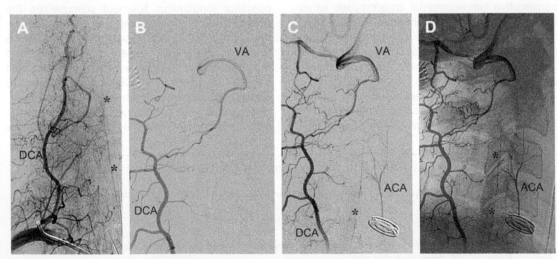

Fig. 2. Right deep cervical artery (DCA) injection, frontal (*A*) and lateral (*B–D*) projections. The anterior spinal artery (*) of the low and mid-cervical spinal cord is supplied from the DCA (*A, C, D*). Collateral reconstitution of the distal right vertebral artery (VA) and anterior cervical artery (ACA) is noted (*B, C, D*).

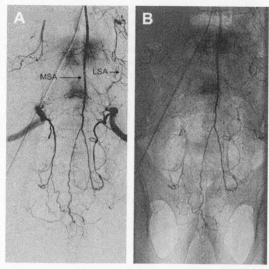

Fig. 3. (*A, B*) Middle sacral artery (MSA) injection, frontal view. Segmental collaterals opacify the lateral sacral (LSA) and internal iliac arteries.

The supply of the spinal dura follows a bilateral segmental distribution, arising from the ventral (intraspinal) division of each dorsal spinal artery.[5] These meningeal vessels supply the nerve root sleeves and give rise to branches ventrally and dorsally within the spinal canal. At the level of the foramen magnum, the ventral dural branches anastomose with dural branches of the ascending pharyngeal artery (**Fig. 7**). The dorsal meningeal arteries likewise anastomose with dural branches of the vertebral, occipital, and unusually, the posterior inferior cerebellar arteries.

VASCULAR SUPPLY TO THE SPINAL CORD

The arteries that supply the neural structures of the spinal canal can be classified into three groups. Small radicular arteries that arise from nearly every segmental level and supply the nerve roots and dural structures locally. If involved in the vascularization of the spinal cord proper, radicular vessels are classified as radiculomedullary (when they supply the anterior spinal artery) or radiculopial (if they contribute to the posterior spinal artery (PSA) and surface vasocorona of the spinal cord).[6-8] They may originate separately or as a common trunk (**Fig. 8**), and follow the nerve root, supplying collaterals to it and the surrounding dura.

The anterior spinal artery is composed of a longitudinal channel located in the anterior median sulcus. It receives contributions at various levels from successive radiculomedullary arteries that arise from the vertebral, ascending and deep cervical, thoracic, and lumbar segmental arteries, respectively. The origin and number of radiculomedullary arteries range from six to ten in adults[9] and include the artery of the lumbar enlargement (arteria radicularis anterior magna—artery of Adamkiewicz), which is the latter most commonly arising from a left thoracic segmental artery between T9 and T12; the artery of the cervical enlargement, which typically arises from vertebral or cervical arteries at the C5 or C6 level; and contribution from the distal vertebral arteries just proximal to the vertebral basilar junction.[10] Angiographically, radiculomedullary branches that contribute to the anterior spinal artery can be recognized by their characteristic "hairpin"

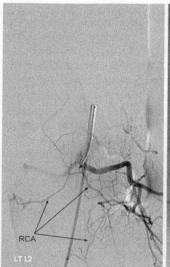
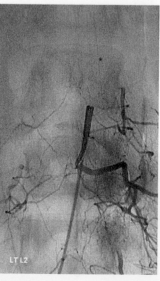

Fig. 4. Retrocorporeal collateral arcade (RCA): characteristically hexagonal network of transverse and longitudinal collateral interconnections within the anterior epidural space. Note collateral reconstitution of adjacent segmental artery (left L1) giving rise to a radiculomedullary branch (*).

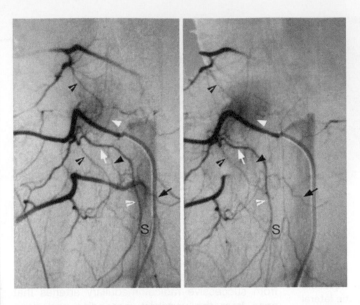

Fig. 5. Extraspinal longitudinal anastomoses between segmental arteries. Radiculopial branch (*white arrowhead*); descending limb of retrocorporeal arcade (*black arrowhead*) anastomosing with contralateral ascending limbs from level below (*black arrow*); pretransverse (*striped black arrowhead*); para-spinous longitudinal arcade (*striped white arrowhead*). S, spinous process.

appearance and midline location. Although the anterior spinal axis is usually a continuous system coursing along the spinal cord within the anterior median sulcus, duplication or fenestrations and discontinuities along its length are not uncommon.

Unlike most arteries, the anterior spinal artery varies in diameter over its length, in a manner matched to the variable metabolic demands of the different spinal cord segments. Caudally, the anterior spinal axis is continuous into the filum terminalis; however, at the conus, it anastomoses with terminal segments of the posterior spinal

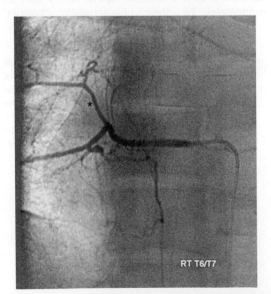

Fig. 6. Enlarged longitudinal collateral (*) coupled with regression of primary T6 segmental artery resulting in common origin of adjacent intercostal arteries.

arteries, forming an identifying arterial "basket." The anterior spinal artery provides two types of tributary branches that supply the spinal cord. Sulcocommisural branches enter the spinal cord parenchyma in the anterior median fissure and supply the anterior two thirds of the cross-sectional area of the spinal cord.[7,8,10] The density of these perforating branches is thought to correspond to the metabolic demand of the underlying gray matter. Consequently, they are particularly numerous throughout the cervical and lumbar enlargements compared with the mid thoracic segments. Circumferential pial branches originate from the anterior spinal artery and exit the anterior median sulcus, coursing laterally to supply the anterolateral surface of the spinal cord before anastomosing with surface branches of the radiculopial circulation.

The surface of the spinal cord can be seen as vascularized by a plexiform vasocorona comprising a collateral network between the paired longitudinal PSA and circumferential pial branches of the anterior spinal artery. Ten to 20 radiculopial arteries contribute to the posterior spinal axis, also forming acute hairpin bifurcations distinguished from the anterior spinal artery by their typical off-midline location. In cases in which spinal pathology distorts the spinal cord, lateral or stereoscopic angiography may clarify any ambiguity. Radially directed perforators (rami perforantes) arise from the surface vasocorona and penetrate to a variable extent the white matter of the spinal funiculi.

The anatomic distribution of spinal arteries establishes three watershed zones: (1) along the longitudinal axis of the upper thoracic spinal cord

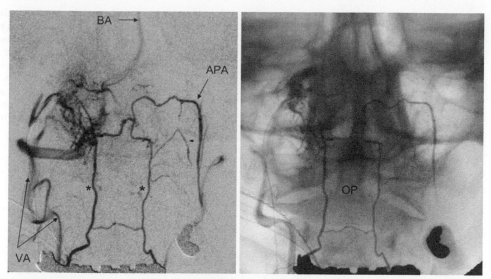

Fig. 7. Ventral dural collaterals between the ascending pharyngeal and vertebral arteries at the level of the craniocervical junction (odontoid arcade). Right ascending pharyngeal artery injection, frontal projection. APA, ascending pharyngeal artery, dural branch; BA, basilar artery; OP, odontoid process; VA, vertebral artery; asterisk (*), ventral dural branch, vertebral artery (C3 level).

between the arteries of the cervical and lumbar enlargements, (2) over the anterolateral surface of the cord between circumferential pial branches of the anterior spinal artery and the posterior spinal arterial arcade, and (3) along the gray/white junction between the intramedullary territories of the central sulcocommisural arteries and the peripheral rami perforantes.

SPINAL VEINS

The venous drainage of the spinal column may be divided into three compartments: (1) the intrinsic and (2) extrinsic venous networks of the spinal cord and (3) the extradural venous plexus.[11] Although the intrinsic venous system is rarely demonstrated angiographically, opacification of

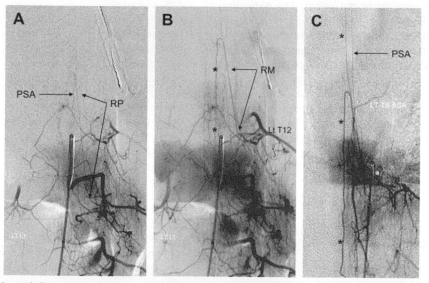

Fig. 8. Radiculomedullary (RM) and radiculopial (RP) branches. (A) Selective left L1 segmental artery injection demonstrates a radiculopial contribution to the posterior spinal artery (PSA). (B) Collateral reconstitution of left T12 pedicle giving rise to radiculomedullary branch (RM) supplying the anterior spinal axis (*) in the same patient. Note the prominent retrocorporeal arcade. (C) Common origin of radiculomedullary and radiculopial braches (different patient) with respective contributions to the anterior (*) and posterior (PSA) spinal arteries.

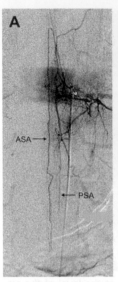
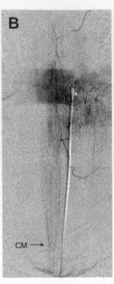
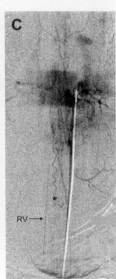

Fig. 9. Selective angiography of thoracic segmental artery with radiculopial and prominent radiculomedullary branch (*A*). ASA, anterior spinal artery; PSA, posterior spinal artery. The vascular "basket" of the conus (CM) is visualized in late arterial phases (*B*). Venous phase image (*C*) reveals radicular (RV) and perimedullary (*) venous channels.

the extrinsic surface spinal cord veins may be seen in delayed phase images under normal conditions during spinal angiography of a prominent radiculomedullary branch (**Fig. 9**). The intramedullary veins, which drain the spinal cord parenchyma, participate in extensive transmedullary anastomoses thought to aid the equalization of venous pressures between ventral and dorsal surfaces of the spinal cord. These parenchymal veins empty into the surface veins of the extrinsic venous network, which includes a rich, superficial venous plexus (particularly dorsally) of perimedullary veins and two longitudinally oriented veins (the posterior and anterior median spinal veins). The extrinsic veins are valveless and empty by way of radicular veins (**Fig. 9**C) into the extradural internal vertebral plexus. In exiting the dura of the thecal sac, functional valves are formed at the level of the radicular veins, preventing retrograde flow (reflux) from the epidural internal vertebral veins into the intrathecal extrinsic venous system of the spinal cord. The internal vertebral veins usually consist of two or more interconnected longitudinal channels situated anteriorly and posteriorly within the spinal epidural space and drain into paravertebral veins through emissary veins at the intervertebral foramina.

REFERENCES

1. Lausjaunias P. Berenstein A. Functional vascular anatomy of the brain, spinal cord and spine. Surgical Neuroangiography, vol. 3. New York: Springer-Verlag; 1990.
2. Chiras J, Morvan G, Merland JJ. The angiographic appearance of the normal intercostal and lumbar arteries: analysis of the anatomic correlation of the lateral branches. J Neuroradiol 1979;6:169–96.
3. Crock HV, Yoshizawa H. Origins of arteries supplying the vertebral column. In: Crock HV, Yoshizawa H, editors. The blood supply of the vertebral column and spinal cord. New York: Springer-Verlag; 1977. p. 1–21.
4. Manelfe C, Djindjian R. Exploration angiographique des angiomes vertebraux. Acta Radiol 1972;13: 818–28 [French].
5. Manelfe C, Lazorthes G, Roulleau J. Arteres de la duremere rachidienne chez l'homme. Acta Radiol 1972;13:829–41 [French].
6. Lazorthes G, Gouaze A, Djindjian R. Vascularisation et circulation de la moelle epiniere. Masson, Paris; 1973.
7. Lazorthes G, Poulhes H, Bastide G. La vascularisation arterielle de la moelle. Neurochirurgie 1958;4: 3–19 [French].
8. Turnbull I. Microvasculature of the human spinal cord. J Neurosurg 1984;35:141–51.
9. Gillilan L. The arterial supply to the human spinal cord. J Comp Neurol 1958;19:110–9.
10. Lazorthes G, Gouaze A, Zadeh O. Arterial vascularization of the spinal cord. J Neurosurg 1971;35: 253–60.
11. Gillilan L. Veins of the spinal cord: anatomic details, suggested clinical applications. Neurology 1970;20: 860–6.

Neurovascular Anatomy: A Practical Guide

Randy Bell, MC, USN[a,b,c], Meryl A. Severson III, MC, USN[a,b], Rocco A. Armonda, MC, USA[a,b],*

KEYWORDS
- Arterial • Venous • Cerebral • Anatomy • Angiography

"The eye only sees what the mind knows."
— Louis Pasteur
"Start at the end and end at the beginning."
— J.R.R. Tolkien
"Sufficiently complicated technology is indistinguishable from magic."
— Arthur Clark

TRAINING THE "MIND'S EYE" IS EQUALLY AS IMPORTANT, IF NOT MORE IMPORTANT, THAN TRAINING ONE'S HANDS

Patterns of normal neurovascular anatomy need to be understood thoroughly before "missing" anatomy or pathologic states can be appreciated. This understanding includes the phenomenon of observing the negative: identifying a missing branch, division, trunk, capillary blush, deep or superficial veins, or venous sinus (**Fig. 1**). As the reference standard of vascular imaging, the dynamic cerebral angiogram facilitates visual acquisition of both overtly present and subtly absent data by providing information that a static two-dimensional picture fails to represent. Coupling these data with rotational, non-subtracted, and subtracted views allows even subtle abnormalities to be detected. During dynamic cerebral angiography, circulation time can be calculated precisely. The speed of venous drainage may indicate pathologic states of rapid filling, as in a fistula, delayed filling, as in increased intracranial pressure, marked venous hypertension, or venous outflow restriction with venous sinus occlusion. In a systematic approach to examining any vascular malformation, it is useful to review the angiogram in a retrograde fashion from late venous phase to arterial phase. Such a review allows the identification of normal venous drainage, capillary blush, and pathological filling of cortical veins during the arterial phase, as well as varix or venous stenosis. Additionally, absent deep central veins are less likely to be overlooked. To reinforce this technique, this article begins at the end of the cerebral circulation and ends at the beginning of the intracranial/intradural circulation. Pathologic processes are demonstrated along this route, as are the limits of various forms of neurovascular imaging. Additional techniques used by the military to image and model three-dimensional targets are demonstrated with photographs of fused-deposition models (see **Fig. 8**). To optimize patient outcomes and to minimize collateral damage, treatment planning includes the review of the noninvasive imaging, the invasive imaging, and the three-dimensional model.

VENOUS SINUSES

The outflow of the cerebral circulation is related to the patency and adequacy of the venous sinuses. Superficially from the jugular bulb retrograde to the sigmoid sinus, the venous sinuses include the transverse sinus, the torcular or confluence of the sinus, and the superior sagittal sinus. The

[a] Department of Neurosurgery, National Capital Consortium, Walter Reed Army Medical Center, 6900 Georgia Ave NW, Washington, DC 20307, USA
[b] Department of Neurosurgery, National Capital Consortium, National Naval Medical Center, 8901 Wisconsin Ave, Bethesda, MD 20889-5600, USA
[c] Department of Neurosurgery, Uniformed Services University of the Health Sciences, 4301 Jones Bridge Road, Bethesda, MD 20814, USA
* Corresponding author.
E-mail address: rocco.armonda@gmail.com (R.A. Armonda).

Neurosurg Clin N Am 20 (2009) 265–278
doi:10.1016/j.nec.2009.04.012
1042-3680/09/$ – see front matter © 2009 Published by Elsevier Inc.

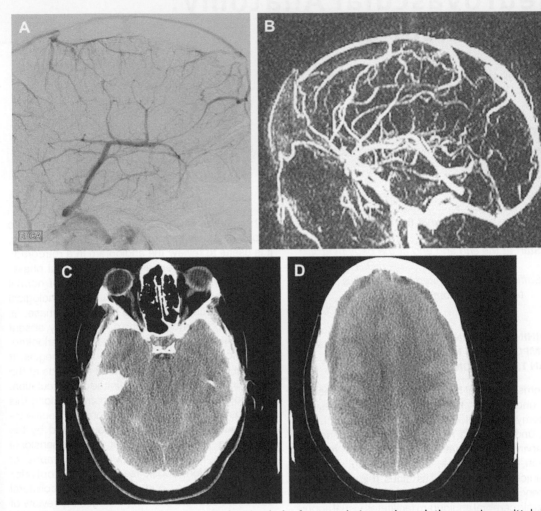

Fig. 1. (*A*) Venous-phase lateral angiogram showing lack of venous drainage through the superior sagittal sinus. (*B*) Magnetic resonance venous image showing misrepresentation of venous flow through the straight sinus and vein of Galen. (*C, D*) CT images of the head showing bilateral chronic subdural hematomas that had resulted in venous sinus compression.

deep venous drainage egresses from the straight sinus, fed by the vein of Galen, which in turn receives output from the internal cerebral veins, inferior sagittal sinus, and the basal veins of Rosenthal. Additional cerebellar venous drainage is carried via the precentral and superior cerebellar veins into the vein of Galen as well as into the tentorial sinuses, which feed into the straight sinus. The brainstem drains through a plexus of rostral to caudal veins that include the pontomesencephalic veins, superior petrosal veins that drain into the superior petrosal sinus or the cavernous sinus. Occasionally, a remnant of the occipital sinus may run in the posterior fossa dura and drain into the marginal sinus surrounding the foramen magnum, which then drains into the paraspinal venous pathways or superiorly towards the torcula.[1] In pathologic states any of these sinuses

can become occluded or overdistended (ie, an arteriovenous fistula), and without valves the direction of blood flow can reverse and result in cortical venous reflux. In the region of the foramen magnum this reflux can result in a variety of presentations from subarachnoid hemorrhage to myelopathy with the transmission of venous hypertension to the spinal cord.

The superior sagittal sinus courses from above the foramen cecum to the torcula, receiving major outflow from the supratentorial cortex. Drainage from the frontal, parietal, and occipital cortex arrives via bridging veins. Named cortical veins include the vein of Trolard from the parietal cortex. This drainage is in balance with drainage from the Sylvian venous system to the sphenoid venous sinus to the cavernous sinus as well as the vein of Labbe drainage from the temporal lobe to the sigmoid sinus. It has been reported that the vein of Labbe is larger on the left, typically dominant, temporal lobe, whereas the vein of Trolard tends to be larger on the nondominant parietal lobe.[2] Occlusion that occurs either traumatically or spontaneously may be tolerated in the anterior third, marginally tolerated in the middle third, and poorly tolerated in the posterior third.[1] Various MRI techniques can misrepresent patency in this and other sinuses. In particular, time-of-flight techniques overestimate occlusion and phase-contrast modes underestimate sinus occlusion and even may indicate sinus patency when catheter-based angiography confirms occlusion (see **Fig. 1**).

The cavernous sinus is the most critical basal venous sinus connecting the intracranial and extracranial circulation. It is a major paired multicompartmental venous sinus and is located on the lateral aspect of the greater wing of the sphenoid. Anterior extracranial input from the facial and angular veins can arrive via the superior and inferior ophthalmic veins. Superior and direct lateral intracranial input arrives from the superficial Sylvian veins to the sphenoparietal sinus to the superior aspect of the cavernous sinus; egress from the medial temporal lobe may drain directly via the uncal vein or middle cerebral vein. The sphenoparietal sinus runs along the lesser wing of the sphenoid and receives input from the frontotemporal lobe via bridging veins from the Sylvian fissure. Connections with the sphenoparietal sinus also include venous drainage from the meningeal, orbital, uncal, and inferior frontal veins. Occasionally, this sinus runs anterior to posterior and is referred to as the "sphenoid-petrosal" sinus. Posterior fossa drainage from the anterior surface of the brainstem and cerebellum arrives via the superior petrosal sinus and inferior petrosal sinus. Because of these connections, two-way traffic may occur in pathologic states through the cavernous carotid, its branches, or the external carotid branches to the cavernous carotid. This two-way traffic may result in orbital, supratentorial, and posterior fossa venous hypertension with multifaceted clinical presentations. In the orbit the most common presentations are chemosis, pulsatile exophthalmos, scleral injection, and increased intraorbital pressures compromising vision. Supratentorial cortical venous reflux can result in intracranial hemorrhage, seizures with temporal lobe venous congestion, and focal neurologic dysfunction including aphasia and memory and cognitive dysfunction. In the posterior fossa this hypertension can manifest as a cerebellar dysfunction with possible hemorrhage and cortical venous distention (**Fig. 2**).

In summary, basal drainage occurs via the cavernous sinus and the basal vein of Rosenthal. Input to the cavernous sinus includes the superficial Sylvian veins, uncal veins, middle cerebral vein, superior ophthalmic veins, inferior ophthalmic veins, and superior petrosal veins with normal outflow through the inferior petrosal sinus and pterygoid plexus in the infratemporal fossa. In pathologic states the venous communication may include direct communication to the basal vein of Rosenthal from an arterialized cavernous sinus.

The basal vein of Rosenthal is formed by the junction of the middle cerebral vein and the inferior striate veins in the anterior perforating substance. The middle cerebral vein receives input from the insular veins and courses around the limen insula before draining into the basal vein of Rosenthal or the cavernous sinus. Its size varies with the size of the superficial Sylvian vein, which, when dominant, dwarfs the middle cerebral vein. The basal vein of Rosenthal has been divided into three segments named in relationship to the cerebral peduncle: the striate segment, the peduncular segment, and the postmesencephalic segment. The third portion, the postmesencephalic segment, drains into the vein of Galen. Drainage from the medial temporal lobe, insula, striatum, midbrain, hypothalamus, and medial orbitofrontal region flows into the basal vein of Rosenthal.[3] In pathologic states marked distention of this vein can cause dominant temporal lobe dysfunction and allow the vein to serve as a reverse pathway from the deep basal compartment to the superficial drainage pathway including the superficial Sylvian vein and vein of Labbe (**Fig. 3**).

The supratentorial deep white matter and lateral ventricular venous outflow converge in the internal cerebral vein in the roof of the third ventricle (**Fig. 4**). The anterior septal and thalamostriate veins join at the venous angle defining the foramen of Monro. Rarely, the anterior septal vein is absent, and the posterior septal veins join the internal cerebral vein at a more distal point in its course, resulting in a misrepresentation of the foramen of Monro. Unlike the ventricular arteries, the veins have a less tortuous and more direct course and are useful in assessing ventricular anatomy.[3]

Drainage of the cerebellum occurs along its three surfaces, suboccipital, petrosal, and tentorial. The vermis and tentorial surface drains through direct connections with the tentorium; vermian drainage also occurs through the superior vermian branch, which drains into the vein of Galen. This branch commonly is coagulated and sectioned to allow microsurgical access to the quadrigeminal cistern and pineal region.

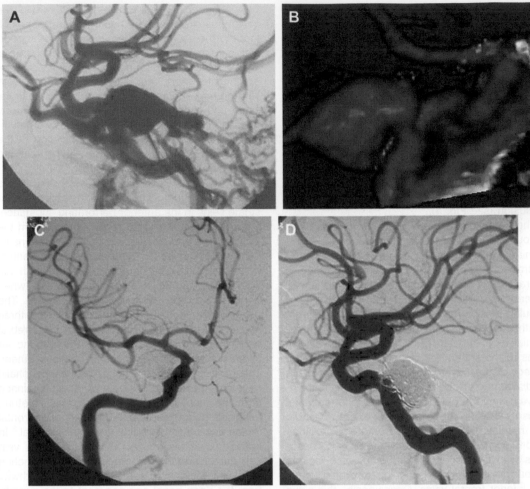

Fig. 2. (*A, B*) Carotid cavernous fistula with cerebellar cortical venous drainage and congestion. (*C, D*) After coil occlusion of the fistula, the cortical venous drainage has resolved.

More superficially located is the inferior vermian vein, which courses from the region of the tonsils paramedian to the straight sinus and is formed by the declival vein and venous contribution from the tonsil. On the petrosal surface, veins are named for their corresponding fissures: the pontomesencephalic and the lateral mesencephalic veins both drain into the superior petrosal vein via the brachial vein and petrosal vein. Alternative drainage pathways may occur toward the vein of Galen through the cerebellomesencephalic fissure and corresponding vein through the precentral cerebellar vein. This vein commonly is displaced in patients who have midline cerebellar masses.[4] The suboccipital surfaces drain via the inferior hemispheric veins, inferior vermian veins that receive input from the tonsillar veins. These tributaries then drain into the transverse or tentorial sinuses. An alternative drainage for these

veins occurs through the cerebellomedullary veins into the petrosal system.[1]

ARTERIAL CIRCULATION: ANTERIOR CIRCULATION

The anterior circulation consists of the supraclinoid carotid and its terminal branches, the anterior cerebral and middle cerebral arteries, and includes the anterior and posterior communicating segments of the circle of Willis. Intracavernous and intrapetrous anastomoses between the external and internal carotid are discussed elsewhere in this issue. The cavernous carotid has three major named branches: the meningohypophyseal trunk, the artery of the inferior cavernous sinus, and the capsular artery (McConell's). The meningohypophyseal trunk arises from the posterior bend of the second intracavernous segment of the carotid artery as described by Rhoton,

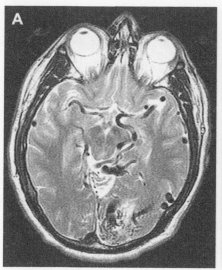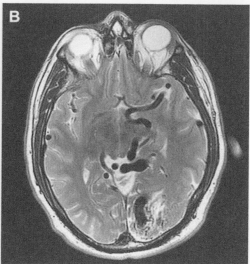

Fig. 3. Progressive venous hypertension with interval increase in the size of the deep venous system. (*A, B*) The markedly enlarged basal vein of Rosenthal and middle cerebral vein drain into the Sylvian vein. Compression and compromise of venous outflow from the dominant left mesial temporal lobe led to multiple memory and neurocognitive disabilities.

contained within Parkinson's triangle which is defined superiorly by the lower boundary of the fourth cranial nerve, inferiorly by the fifth cranial nerve, and posteriorly the slope of the dorsum sella and the clivus. The three major branches of the meningohypophyseal trunk are the tentorial artery (Bernasconi-Cassinari), the inferior hypophyseal artery, and the dorsal meningeal artery. The tentorial artery is the largest and has connections with the contralateral tentorial artery converging on the incisural apex.[5] It is markedly enlarged in selected cases of tentorial dural arteriovenous malformations (AVMs) and meningiomas.

Ophthalmic Artery

In most patients the ophthalmic artery originates from the superomedial aspect of the internal carotid artery (ICA) just above the dural ring. Other less common points of origination include the intracavernous carotid artery (8% of cases) possibly representing a remnant dorsal primitive ophthalmic artery, the anterior cerebral artery representing a remnant ventral ophthalmic artery, and the middle meningeal artery typically coursing into the orbit via the optic canal beneath the optic nerve but in rare cases coursing through the optic strut. The artery then rolls upward from a lateral to a medial direction, coursing over the optic nerve in 85% of cases. Variations in this pattern and its neuroendovascular consequences have been reviewed elegantly and discussed by Perrini and

colleagues.[6] The ophthalmic branches can be organized into four groups: ocular, orbital, extraorbital, and dural. The ocular group includes the central retinal artery and the ciliary arteries supplying the retina and choroid. The orbital group includes the lacrimal and muscular branches. The extraorbital group includes the supraorbital, anterior and posterior ethmoidal, palpebral, dorsal nasal, and supratrochlear arteries. The dural group includes the recurrent meningeal and deep meningeal branches. The ethmoidal and lacrimal branches also contribute to the ophthalmic artery.

Within the first segment of the ophthalmic artery the first terminal branch, the central retinal artery, arises at the "bayonet" point of the ophthalmic artery and continues forward as the artery courses over the nerve. The next branches are the posterior ciliary arteries. Occasionally, the central retinal artery may share a common trunk with the posterior ciliary and muscular branches. Less commonly, the ophthalmic artery may pass from above the optic nerve to below it; in this case the order of the branching is reversed, with the posterior ciliary arteries branching first and the central retinal artery branching second branch (also known as the second segment). The second segment of the ophthalmic artery then gives rise to the posterior ciliary arteries (supplying the choroid), and the lacrimal artery coursing with the lacrimal nerve to the lacrimal gland superomedially towards the lateral rectus. The third segment then gives rise to the anterior and posterior ethmoidal arteries, which supply the ethmoid

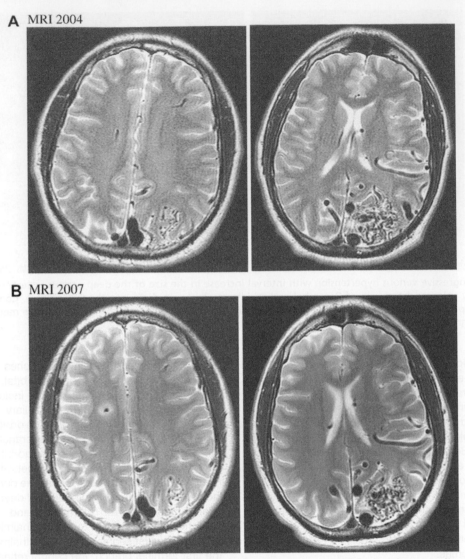

A MRI 2004

B MRI 2007

Fig. 4. MRIs performed (*A*) in 2004 and (*B*) in 2007 show the interval increase of T2 signal surrounding a contralateral vein located in the right hemisphere white matter draining into the lateral ventricle.

sinuses, nasal cavity, and septum. The anterior ethmoidal artery tends to be larger and to be an independent branch from the ophthalmic artery. It also continues anteriorly as the artery of the falx cerebri or anterior falx artery. This branch usually is bilaterally involved in cases of anterior cranial dural AVMs. The posterior ethmoidal sends branches to the posterior and medial portions of the anterior cranial fossa. The terminal branch coursing through the orbit is the supraorbital artery, which anastomoses with the superficial temporal artery along the superior temporal line.

Additional anastomoses with the external carotid system can exist though several routes. The angular branch of the facial artery may anastomose with the nasal artery from the terminal portion of the ophthalmic artery. The infraorbital, anterior, and deep temporal arteries from the internal maxillary artery can connect with the inferior lacrimal territory, and the recurrent middle meningeal artery may connect with the anterior branch of the middle meningeal artery. This anastomosis between the lacrimal artery and the recurrent branch of the middle meningeal artery is seen most commonly when the lacrimal artery originates from the ophthalmic artery. These connections put the ophthalmic artery at risk during epistaxis or other embolizations of the internal maxillary artery.[6]

Posterior Communicating Artery

Arising from the posteromedial aspect of the supraclinoid carotid artery in its normal configuration, the posterior communicating artery (PComA) completes the posterior connection of the circle of Willis at the posterior cerebral artery (PCA) at the junction of P1-P2. In 22% of cases it is larger than the PCA or fails to fuse, remaining a fetal PCA connection to the occipital lobe. The normal (small-sized) PComA courses posteromedially, joining the PCA above and medial to the oculomotor nerve. In a fetal configuration it courses further laterally, above or lateral to the oculomotor nerve, where it continues as the PCA. Its largest branch, usually from the middle third of the PComA, is the premammillary artery (also known as the "anterior thalamoperforating artery"), which gives rise to perforating branches. A group of anterior perforating branches supply the posterior limb of the internal capsule, the anterior third of the optic tract, whereas the posterior perforators penetrate the rostral midbrain and the subthalamic nucleus. Occlusion of the branches may result in diencephalic infarct as well as contralateral hemiballism with subthalamic nucleus infarct.[7] Although the PComA can be occluded safely when collateral circulation to these perforators is preserved, a resulting capsular infarct may result in rare cases when the collateral supply is inadequate. Additionally, in the presence of PComA aneurysm, persistent retrograde filling may occur, allowing aneurysm growth or re-rupture. In PComA aneurysms when the PComA has a proximal intracranial origin, it may be necessary to obtain proximal control of the cervical ICA during surgery (**Fig. 5**).

Anterior Choroidal Artery

The anterior choroidal artery (AChA) originates from the posterolateral aspect of the ICA, coursing medially beneath the optic tract, lateral to the crus cerebri, into the internal choroidal fissure at the uncus. Alternative origins include the middle cerebral artery (MCA) (11.7%), the PComA (6.7%), and the ICA bifurcation (3.3%). The AChA is divided into the cisternal and choroidal or plexal portions. The cisternal portion supplies the optic tract and optic radiations, the middle third of the cerebral peduncle, the temporal lobe, the posterior limb of the internal capsule, the globus pallidus, and the lateral geniculate body. The choroidal point is the portion of the AChA entering the temporal horn of the lateral ventricle. In up to 16% of patients, however, the medial perforating branches may arise from the ventricular or plexal segments. Of note, 57% of the hippocampal arteries arise from both the PCA and AChA; only 3% arise from the AChA alone. Occlusion of the AChA usually is associated with contralateral

hemiplegia, hemianesthesia, and hemianopia. Hemiplegia and hemianesthesia result from infarction of the posterior two thirds of the posterior limb of the internal capsule and of the middle third of the cerebral peduncle. Homonymous hemianopia results from the interruption of supply to the occipital cortex. Incongruous visual fields occur more commonly with lesion of the lateral geniculate body. These deficits are not predictably reproducible. In fact, in 1954 Cooper[8,9] reported the resolution of Parkinson symptoms, in particular rigidity and tremor, with preservation of voluntary motor function likely caused by ischemic necrosis of the globus pallidus. Preservation of anastomosis via the lateral geniculate body in the choroid plexus is postulated to have allowed preservation of the voluntary motor function.

Middle Cerebral Artery

The MCA courses as the terminal bifurcation of the ICA. It is divided into four segments and has a variable length, course, and branch configuration. The M1 (sphenoidal) segment is from the ICA terminus to the limen insula. The M2 (insular) segment occurs from this point to the second turn of the artery at the circular sulcus, where the M3 (opercular) portions begin. These segments continue until the branches course over the frontal, temporal, and parietal cortical surfaces to become the M4 (cortical) branches. The course of the M1 segment may parallel the sphenoid wing or curve anteriorly or posteriorly. This portion gives rise to the anterior temporal branch inferiorly and also gives rise to multiple posteriorly and superiorly directed lateral lenticulostriate branches (**Fig. 6**). In some cases the MCA bifurcates proximally and the superior trunk then courses anteriorly. This early bifurcation also is associated with a higher rate of microsurgical complications. Anatomically, this early frontal branch gives rise to lateral lenticulostriate vessels and is less tolerant of temporary artery clipping.[10]

The MCA trifurcation typically is a series of dual bifurcations rather than a true trifurcation. Four different patterns have been classically described: a single dominant trunk, bifurcation, trifurcation, and quadrification. The bifurcation into an anterior division and posterior division is most common; of these bifurcations, 32% are inferiorly dominant, 28% are superiorly dominant, and 18% are equally divided. In rare cases the MCA may originate from the anterior cerebral artery or be duplicated with a parallel branch arising from the A1-2 segment coursing through the Sylvian fissure to the cortex. MCA cortical branches include the orbitofrontal artery and the operculofrontal artery, with anterior

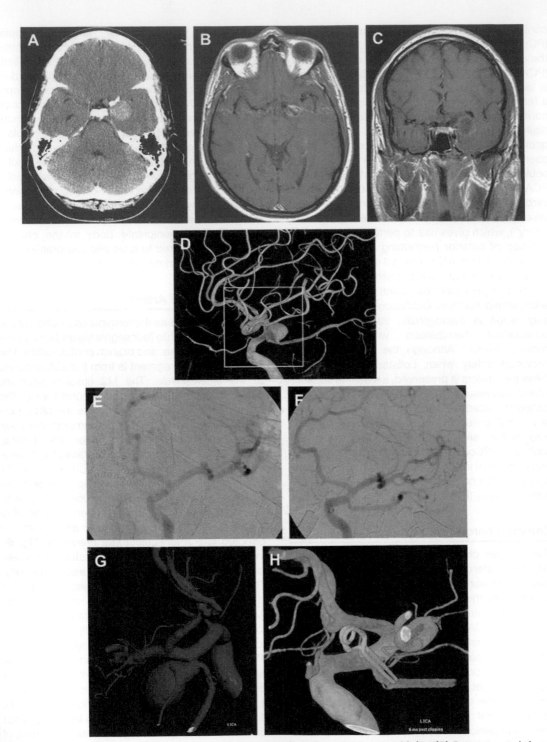

Fig. 5. (A–C) CT and MR images showing a round mass in the left mesial temporal lobe. (D) Reconstructed three-dimensional (3D) rotational angiogram reveals a large aneurysm arising from the origin of the left posterior communicating artery. (E) Intraoperative angiogram shows complete occlusion of the parent vessel with (F) subsequent re-establishment of flow and obliteration of the aneurysm after clip repositioning. (G) Preoperative and (H) postoperative reconstructed 3D rotational angiogram shows continued obliteration of the aneurysm with preservation of the parent vessel. Note the anterior choroidal artery arising just distal to the origin of the posterior communicating artery.

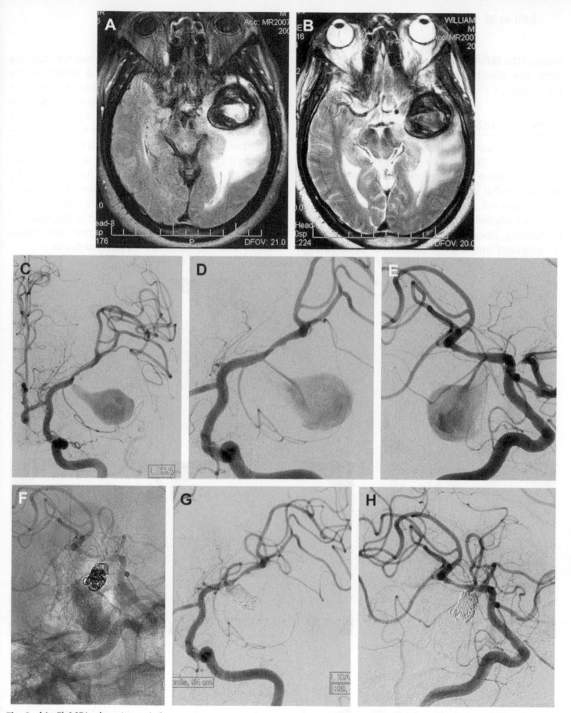

Fig. 6. (*A*, *B*) MRIs showing a left anterior temporal mass with significant edema. (*C–E*) Digitally subtracted angiography images showing a partially thrombosed giant left MCA aneurysm. Note the upward displacement of the left MCA as well as the medial deflection of the left anterior temporal artery. (*F–H*) Digitally subtracted images showing coils within the aneurysm and isolation from the circulation. The mass effect from the aneurysm is still present, however. (*Courtesy of* Dr. William O. Bank, Director of Interventional Neuroradiology, Washington Hospital Center, Washington, DC.)

frontal branches. The anterior frontal branches include the pre-Rolandic, central, post-Rolandic, anterior parietal, posterior parietal, and the angular arteries. The posterior division includes the temporal, polar, anterior temporal, middle temporal, posterior temporal, and temporal occipital arteries. Normal flow and anatomy of these distal branches may be distorted in various pathologic states (**Figs. 7** and **8**). The Sylvian Triangle is formed by a line coursing through the fissure at the apex of the MCA branches to the Sylvian Point and from the sulcus limitans directed to the MCA bifurcation.

Anterior Cerebral Artery

The anterior cerebral artery, the terminal segment of the ICA, is divided into five segments. The first segment before the communicating segment gives rise to medial perforating branches that course behind the A1 segment. The recurrent artery of Heubner courses from the A1-2 junction and runs posteriorly, abutting the gyrus rectus. Rarely, the A1 segment may course beneath or even through the optic nerve. This infraoptic course can be appreciated on angiography by a notch in the angiogram in the A1 segment. Occasionally, this arterial course will be associated with a lack of an interhemispheric fissure seen as abnormal gyral segmentation on MRI.[11] Otherwise the A1 courses over the optic nerve and chiasm junction medially before it continues to the anterior communication segment and superiorly (as the A2 designation) beneath the corpus callosum. Around the genu of the corpus callosum, the artery bifurcates, giving rise to the pericallosal branch along the body of the corpus callosum and to the callosomarginal artery over the cingulate sulcus and gyrus.

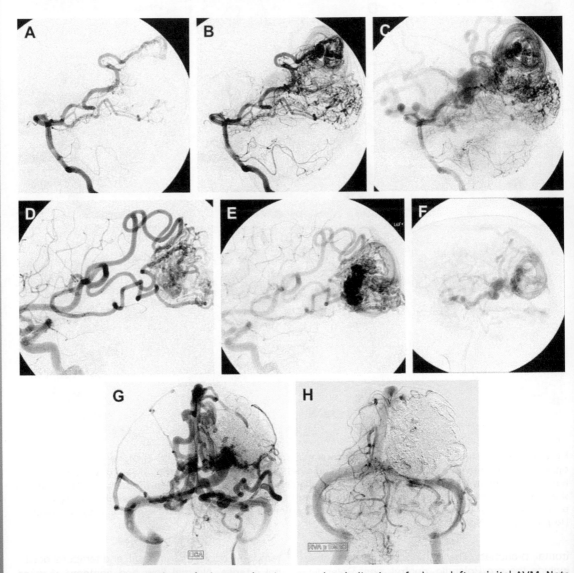

Fig. 7. Digital subtraction angiography images showing staged embolization of a large left occipital AVM. Note that the AVM fills robustly from both the posterior (*A–C*) and anterior (*D–F*) circulations. Anteroposterior venous-phase images after (*G*) ICA and (*H*) VA injection with marked venous hypertension and large varix that drains into the deep system.

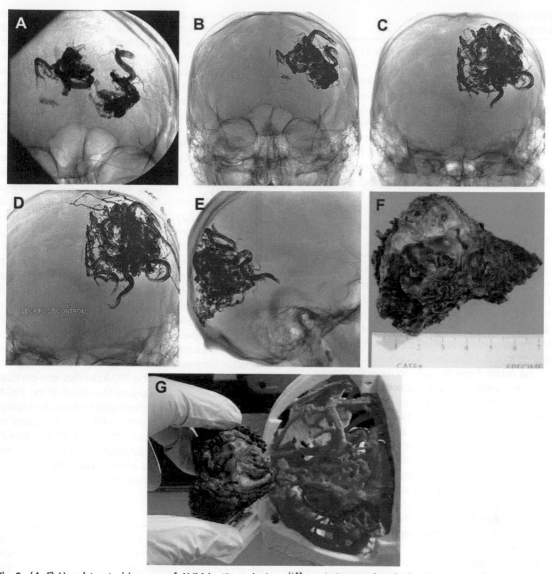

Fig. 8. (*A–E*) Unsubtracted images of AVM in **Fig. 4** during different stages of embolization. Note the sequential increase of radiopaque embolic material. (*F*) The AVM measuring approximately 7 cm from cortical to deep component has been resected. (*G*) Comparison of the specimen is made with a 3D fused deposition model constructed preoperatively. These models are highly useful for preoperative planning. They allow the surgeon to see and manipulate the malformation and the surrounding vascular structures easily in three dimensions.

The AComA region has a large number of variations that can include duplication of the communicating branch, a variety of fenestrations, a primary balanced trunk, or lateral dominant A1 segments. At the level of the AComA there may be one to three trunks forming the A2 branches as well as the recurrent artery of Heubner. Occlusion of this critical branch may lead to hemiparesis with upper extremity and facial manifestations involving the anterior limb of the internal capsule. In rare cases an undivided or azygous ACA occurs as a single midline vessel from the confluence of the A1, ACAs, and paired A2 vessels. This undivided ACA then divides into bilateral pericallosal and callosomarginal arteries distal to the genu of the corpus callosum. Most commonly this variant occurs with a central accessory ACA dominant to the two parallel branches. This central ACA variant arises from a retained, dominant median artery of the corpus callosum. Rare aneurysms are nonsaccular, without a discrete neck, and require clip reconstruction. It is postulated that aneurysms occurring here have twice the degree of hemodynamic stress.[12]

POSTERIOR CIRCULATION
Vertebral Arteries

The blood supply to the contents of the posterior fossa is entirely from the vertebrobasilar complex.[13] Congenital anomalies, traumatic injuries, and cerebrovascular disease affecting this complex thus can have devastating neurologic consequences. The vertebral arteries (VAs) give rise to this important vascular tree and most commonly are the first branch from the subclavian arteries. The left VA is dominant in 60% of individuals[14] and originates from the aortic arch in 0.5% of individuals.[15] The right VA is hypoplastic in 10%, the left VA is hypoplastic in 5%,[16] and the VA ends in the posterior inferior cerebellar artery (PICA) in 0.2%.[13]

The VA is divided into four segments: the extraosseous, V1; the foraminal, V2; the extraspinal, V3; and the intradural, V4.[17] V1 extends from its origin to the entrance of the foramen transversarium of the sixth cervical vertebra. The VA enters C6 in 90% of individuals, C5 in 7%, and C7 in 3%.[18] V2 extends to the axis where the artery turns laterally to exit the foramen. V3 encompasses the exit of the artery from the axis to its entrance into the foramen magnum. V4 extends from the point where it pierces the dura to its junction with the contralateral VA at the vertebral confluens, which demarcates the pontomedullary junction.[16] Fenestration of the VA, most commonly located at the V4 segment, is associated with vascular malformations and intracranial aneurysms.[19]

The branches of the VA are broadly divided into cervical, meningeal, and intracranial groups.[20] The cervical branches include the muscular and spinal branches supplying the deep cervical musculature as well as the spinal cord, its meninges, and the vertebral bodies.[13] Muscular branches may anastomose with the occipital and ascending pharyngeal arteries from the external carotid artery,[13,21] and the neurosurgeon and interventionalist must be aware of possible anastomoses when embolizing dural arteriovenous fistulas and AVMs in this location. In these instances aggressive embolization of external carotid pedicles can lead to VA territorial infarcts. These anastomoses also may provide important collateral blood flow to the posterior fossa in cases of proximal VA occlusion.[13] The anterior meningeal artery arises at C2 and supplies the dura of the foramen magnum. The posterior meningeal branch supplies the falx cerebelli and the occipital dura.[13] Intracranial branches of the VA include the anterior and posterior spinal arteries, small perforators, and the PICA.[13]

The PICA is the largest branch and most commonly arises intradurally. It provides blood supply to the suboccipital cerebellar surface as well as the tonsils, inferior vermis, and inferior fourth ventricle.[14] It may have an extradural origin in 5% of individuals[20] and may be as low as C1 or C2.[13] Anomalous origin of the PICA from ICA is associated with increased risk of intracranial aneurysm,[22,23] as is a duplicated PICA.[24] When the PICA is developmentally absent, the anterior inferior cerebellar artery (AICA) often is enlarged, supplying its normal territory as well as that of the missing PICA;[21] this condition often is termed an "AICA-PICA trunk." The PICA has five segments;[25] the first three must be preserved during intervention (surgery or endovascular), but the last two may be taken with little risk of neurologic compromise.[26] The anterior medullary segment extends from the PICA origin to the inferior olivary prominence; its branches supply the ventral medulla. The lateral medullary segment extends to the origin of cranial nerves IX, X, and XI along the lateral brainstem, which it supplies. The tonsillomedullary segment extends to the tonsillar midportion and on lateral angiography is seen as the caudal loop of the PICA. The tonsillomedullary segment is seen as the cranial loop on angiography. Finally, the PICA divides into cortical branches. The three largest branches of the PICA include the choroidal artery arising from the cranial loop. The choroidal point, defined as the apex of the cranial loop, defines the floor of the fourth ventricle on lateral angiography. The tonsillohemispheric artery and the inferior vermian artery are the other major branches.[16]

Basilar Artery

The basilar artery is formed by the confluence of the VAs at the pontomedullary junction. In cases of incomplete fusion during development, the basilar artery may be fenestrated at its origin.[13] Aneurysms can form at the site of fenestration.[19] The artery then courses ventral to the brainstem to the pontomesencephalic junction, where it bifurcates into the PCAs in the interpeduncular cistern or posterior portion of the suprasellar cistern.[13] In 70% of cases, the level of the bifurcation is even with or above the posterior clinoid.[27] Anteriorly pointing basilar summit aneurysms above the posterior clinoid are easier to access surgically than are low-lying or posteriorly pointing aneurysms.[14] In elderly patients and in patients who have hypertension or cerebrovascular disease, the basilar artery often follows an ectatic course. Branches include the AICAs, the superior cerebellar arteries, the PCAs, the labyrinthine arteries, and as many as 17 pontine perforators.[28] Perforating vessels may be paramedian and short or circumferential and long. Paramedian vessels penetrate the anterior surface of the brainstem, whereas the circumferential arteries penetrate more laterally; perfusion by both groups respects the midline.[14] The labyrinthine artery originates from the AICA in 45% of individuals, from the superior cerebellar artery in 25%, and from the basilar artery itself in 16%,[13] and courses into the internal acoustic meatus.[29]

The AICA originates from the rostral basilar artery, traveling through the cerebellopontine angle near cranial nerves VII and VIII.[21] It is a single vessel in 72% of individuals, is duplicated in 26%, and is triplicated in 2%.[30] It provides blood supply to the petrosal surface of the cerebellum.[14] The AICA sends branches to the internal acoustic meatus via the labyrinthine artery, the foramen of Luschka, and the flocculus.[31] The caudal trunk anastomoses with the PICA, and the rostral trunk anastomoses with the superior cerebellar artery.[18]

The superior cerebellar artery originates inferior to cranial nerve III,[21] travels in the perimesencephalic cistern,[32] and commonly is duplicated. It supplies the tentorial surface of the cerebellum as well as the superior vermis, upper pons, and lower midbrain.[14] At the origin, the superior cerebellar arteries are separated from the PCAs by cranial nerve III, and distally these vessels are separated by the tentorium.[13] The superior cerebellar artery is composed of four segments: the anterior and lateral pontomesencephalics, the cerebellomesencephalic, and the cortical segment.[18,31]

Posterior Cerebral Arteries

The PCAs originate from the distal basilar artery and have four named segments: the precommunicating segment, P1; the ambient segment, P2; the quadrigeminal segment, P3; and the calcarine segment, P4.[33] They supply the posterior cerebral hemispheres, a portion of the midbrain and thalamus, and the choroid plexus of the lateral and third ventricles.[34] P1 extends from the PCA origin to the junction with the PComA. Approximately 33% of the time the PCA is termed "fetal," because the diameter of P1 is less than that of the PComA and the PCA fills predominantly from the ICA.[34] P1 branches include the thalamoperforators, which pass through the interpeduncular fossa and penetrate the posterior perforated substance.[33]

P2 extends to the posterior border of the midbrain traveling in the crural (P2A) and ambient (P2P) cisterns.[34] It gives rise to the thalamogeniculate and peduncular perforators, the posterior choroidal arteries, and the anterior and posterior

temporal arteries.[33] The medial posterior choroidal artery enters the roof of the third ventricle, passes through the foramen of Monro, and supplies the choroid plexus of the lateral ventricle. The lateral posterior choroidal arteries pass through the choroidal fissure to the choroid of the atrium and lateral horn and anastomose with branches of the AChA. The anterior temporal artery arises from P2 and passes under the hippocampal gyrus to anastomose with branches of the anterior temporal artery from the MCA. The posterior temporal artery also arises from P2 and runs posterolaterally providing blood supply to the inferior temporal and occipital lobes.[33]

The P3 segment extends to the entrance of the calcarine fissure, and P4 is the termination of the artery into its cortical branches as it enters the fissure.[33] The terminal branches include the parieto-occipital and calcarine arteries supplying the visual cortex, the splenial arteries supplying the posterior corpus callosum, and the lateral occipital artery supplying the inferior temporal lobe.[33] To aid in identifying these vessels on lateral angiography, a line is traced over the straight sinus seen in the venous phase. Vessels seen below this line in the arterial phase are lateral and therefore are temporal cortical branches; the first vessel superior to the straight sinus is the calcarine artery deep in the calcarine fissure, and the parieto-occipital artery follows a posterosuperior course in the parieto-occipital fissure.[35]

REFERENCES

1. Matsushima T, Rhoton AL Jr, de Olivera E, et al. Microsurgical anatomy of the veins of the posterior fossa. J Neurosurg 1983;59(1):63–105.

2. Andrews BT, Dujovny M, Mirchandani HG, et al. Microsurgical anatomy of the venous drainage into the superior sagittal sinus. Neurosurgery 1989; 24(4):514–20.

3. Morris P. The venous system. In: Practical neuroangiography. 2nd edition. Philadelphia: Lippincott Williams & Wilkins; 2007. p. 271–88.

4. Huang YP, Wolf BS. Angiographic features of brainstem tumors and differential diagnosis from fourth ventricle tumors. Am J Roentgenol Radium Ther Nucl Med 1970;110:1–30.

5. Van Lovern HR, Keller JT, EL-Kalliny M, et al. The Dolenc technique for cavernous sinus exploration (cadaveric prosection). J Neurosurg 1991;74: 837–44.

6. Perrini P, Cardia A, Fraser K, et al. A microsurgical study of the anatomy and course of the ophthalmic artery and its potential dangerous anastomoses. J Neurosurg 2007;106:142–50.

7. Rhoton AL. Cranial anatomy and surgical approaches. Schaumberg (IL): Lippincott Williams & Wilkins; 2003.

8. Cooper IS. Surgical alleviation of parkinsonism: effect of occlusion of the anterior choroidal artery. J Am Geriatr Soc 1954;2:691–718.

9. Cooper IS. Surgical occlusion of the anterior choroidal artery in parkinsonsim. Surg Gynecol Obstet 1954;99:207–19.

10. Ulm AJ, Fautheree GL, Tanriover N, et al. Microsurgical and angiographic anatomy of middle cerebral artery aneurysms: prevalence and significance of early branching aneurysms. Neurosurgery 2008;62: ONS344–53.

11. McLaughlin N, Bojanowski MW. Infraoptic course of anterior cerebral arteries associated with abnormal gyral segmentation. J Neurosurg 2007;107:430–4.

12. Auguste KI, Ware ML, Lawton MT. Nonsaccular aneurysms of the azygous anterior cerebral artery. Neurosurg Focus 2004;17(5):E12.

13. Osborn AG. The vertebrobasilar system. In: Diagnostic cerebral angiography. 2nd edition. Philadelphia: Lippincott Williams & Wilkins; 1999. p. 173–94.

14. Morris P. The arteries of the posterior fossa. In: Practical neuroangiography. 2nd edition. Philadelphia: Lippincott Williams & Wilkins; 2007. p. 253–70.

15. Osborn AG. The aortic arch and great vessels. In: Diagnostic cerebral angiography. 2nd edition. Philadelphia: Lippincott Williams & Wilkins; 1999. p. 3–29.

16. Greenberg MS. Anatomy. In: Handbook of neurosurgery. New York: Thieme; 2006. p. 68–93.

17. Subclavian system of arteries. In: Williams PL, editor. Gray's anatomy. 38th edition. New York: Churchill Livingstone; 1995. p. 1529–34.

18. Lang J. Clinical anatomy of the posterior cranial fossa and its foramina. New York: Thieme; 1991. p. 15–46.

19. Tran-Dinh HD. Duplication of the vertebro-basilar system. Australas Radiol 1991;35:220–4.

20. Newton TH, Mani RL. The vertebral artery. Book 2. In: Newton TH, Potts DG, editors, Radiology of the skull and brain: angiography, vol. 2. St Louis (MO): Mosby; 1974. p. 1659–709.

21. Grand W, Hopkins LN. Vertebral and basilar arteries. In: Grand W, Hopkins LN, editors. Vasculature of the brain and cranial base. New York: Thieme; 1999. p. 161–79.

22. Manabe H, Oda N, Ishii M, et al. The posterior inferior cerebellar artery originating from the internal carotid artery, associated with multiple aneurysms. Neuroradiology 1991;33:513–5.

23. Ahuja A, Graves VB, Crosby DL, et al. Anomalous origin of the posterior inferior cerebellar artery from the internal carotid artery. AJNR Am J Neuroradiol 1992;13:1625–6.

24. Lesley WS, Rajab MH, Case RS. Double origin of the posterior inferior cerebellar artery: association with intracranial aneurysm on catheter angiography. AJR Am J Roentgenol 2007;189(4):893–7.

25. Lister JR, Rhoton AL, Matsushima T, et al. Microsurgical anatomy of the posterior inferior cerebellar artery. Neurosurgery 1982;10:170–99.

26. Getch CC, O'Shaughnessy BA, Bendock BR, et al. Surgical management of intracranial aneurysms involving the posterior inferior cerebellar artery. Contemp Neurosurg 2004;26(9):1–7.

27. Caruso G, Vincentelli F, Giudicelli G, et al. Perforating branches of the basilar bifurcation. J Neurosurg 1990;73(2):259–65.

28. Torche M, Mahmood A, Araujo R, et al. Microsurgical anatomy of the lower basilar artery. Neurol Res 1992; 14(3):259–62.

29. Brunsteins DB, Ferreri AJM. Microsurgical anatomy of VII and VIII cranial nerves and related arteries in the cerebellopontine angle. Surg Radiol Anat 1990; 12:259–65.

30. Martin RG, Grant JL, Peace D, et al. Microsurgical relationships of the anterior inferior cerebellar artery and the facial-vestibulocochlear nerve complex. Neurosurgery 1980;6:483–507.

31. Matsuno H, Rhoton AL, Peace D. Microsurgical anatomy of the posterior fossa cisterns. Neurosurgery 1988;23:58–80.

32. Armonda RA, Rosenwasser RH. Vascular anatomy of the central nervous system. In: Jafar JJ, Awad IA, Rosenwasser RH, editors. Vascular malformations of the central nervous system. Philadelphia: Lippincott Williams & Wilkins; 1999. p. 19–45.

33. Osborn AG. Posterior cerebral artery. In: Diagnostic cerebral angiography. 2nd edition. Philadelphia: Lippincott Williams & Wilkins; 1999. p. 153–71.

34. Rhoton AL. The cerebrum. Neurosurgery 2007; 61(SHC Suppl 1):SHC37–SHC119.

35. Morris P. The posterior cerebral artery. In: Practical neuroangiography. 2nd edition. Philadelphia: Lippincott Williams & Wilkins; 2007. p. 226–39.

Intracranial Collateral Anastomoses: Relevance to Endovascular Procedures

Adnan H. Siddiqui, MD, PhD[a],*, Peng R. Chen, MD[b]

KEYWORDS

- Complication avoidance
- Extracranial-to-intracranial anastomoses
- Intracranial anastomoses • Intracranial collateralization
- Neurointerventional procedures • Vascular anatomy

Endovascular strategies for addressing intracranial and extracranial disease continue to gain momentum. These techniques are limited principally by technology and imagination. As newer devices and implements are introduced to the endovascular surgeon, more diseases previously construed to be the realm of open surgery or untreatable are becoming amenable to endovascular interventions. Because of the nature of endovascular procedures, with liquid agents, flow-directed therapies, and embolic materials, it is critical for the endovascular surgeon to be aware of the collaterals that exist between the vessels being embolized and other critical collaterally connected vessels, occlusion of which may result in undesirable outcomes. Similarly, for other occasions, such collaterals may provide unique conduits that may afford access in novel ways to the intracranial or extracranial circulation. The understanding of these collaterals is best undertaken with an initial understanding of the development of the cranial vasculature. The rich anastomotic connections and interlinked development shed great light and provide a firm basis for understanding the cranial collaterals. The collateral circulation may be divided by collaterals between extracranial and intracranial systems and collaterals between the internal carotid and vertebrobasilar (VB) systems. This article provides a brief overview of cranial vascular development, followed by specific clinically relevant examples of extracranial and intracranial anastomoses and the internal carotid artery (ICA) and VB anastomoses.

CRANIAL VASCULAR EMBRYOLOGY

The cranial vasculature begins with the development of a vascular supply to the paired pharyngeal arches. This supply develops as vascular arches that emanate from the ventral aortic sac connect with the paired dorsal aortae. Each pharyngeal arch gets its own vascular arch. These vascular arches then develop and regress in rostrocaudal fashion. The pharyngeal arches become apparent at approximately 3 to 4 weeks' gestation. The pharyngeal arches develop plexiform vascular channels that ultimately connect the ventral aortic sac with the paired dorsal aortae, forming the vascular arch. The first arch gives rise to the primitive stapedial artery, whereas the second gives rise to the hyoid artery. These arches then regress and coalesce to form the primitive hyoidostapedial artery. These vessels are critical to the vascular development of the skull base. This primitive branch follows the three divisions of the trigeminal

---

[a] Department of Neurosurgery, School of Medicine and Biomedical Sciences, Millard Fillmore Gates Hospital, Kaleida Health, State University of New York, University at Buffalo, 3 Gates Circle, Buffalo, NY 14209, USA
[b] Department of Neurosurgery, University of Texas at Houston, Houston, TX, USA
* Corresponding author.
E-mail address: adnan.h.siddiqui@gmail.com (A.H. Siddiqui).

Neurosurg Clin N Am 20 (2009) 279–296
doi:10.1016/j.nec.2009.04.013
1042-3680/09/$ – see front matter © 2009 Published by Elsevier Inc.

nerve such that one trunk that develops along the mandibular division becomes the adult internal maxillary artery; the superior trunk becomes the middle meningeal artery and contributes to the ophthalmic artery. The primitive maxillary artery develops as the meningohypophyseal trunk, whereas the third division becomes the cortico-tympanic branch, which communicates with the ICA in the petrous canal (**Fig. 1**). An embryologic dorsal ophthalmic artery regresses to become the inferolateral trunk, rarely staying on as a cavernous origin to the adult ophthalmic artery.[1] The third vascular arch on either side becomes the cervical ICA, eventually incorporating parts of the dorsal aortae bilaterally to form more cranial sections up the posterior communicating artery (PCoA) segment. From the third arch sprouts the external carotid artery (ECA) trunk, which anastomoses with the primitive hyoidostapedial artery branches to complete the ECA circuitry. Additionally, a pair of plexiform networks, called the "ventral pharyngeal arteries," develops early on and connects to the hyoidostapedial trunk. These ventral-pharyngeal networks form before the development of the ECA trunk, eventually mostly regressing, but retaining parts that allow for anastomoses between the ascending pharyngeal and caroticotympanic arteries.

The posterior circulation develops in parallel, first appearing toward the beginning of the fifth gestational week as paired dorsal longitudinal neural arteries. These eventually form the intracranial vertebral arteries (VA) and basilar artery. Further caudally, a plexiform network of the cervical intersegmental arteries anastomoses to form the paired VAs. As these channels continue to develop, they reliably develop anastomotic connections with the ICAs, forming the trigeminal, otic, hypoglossal, and proatlantal intersegmental connections (**Fig. 2**). The seventh cervical interseg-mental artery coalesces with the right fourth vascular arch (the right aortic arch) to form the prox-imal part of the subclavian artery and from it origi-nates the VA. On the left side, the seventh cervical intersegmental artery coalesces with the left aortic arch (distal fourth arch–true adult aortic arch) to form the proximal left subclavian artery and from it originates the left VA (**Fig. 3**). By 6 weeks' gesta-tion, the cranial-most end of the ICAs has divided into rostral and caudal divisions. Although the rostral division forms the anterior, middle, and ante-rior choroidal arteries, the caudal division fuses with the dorsal longitudinal neural arteries to form the PCoA. This results in eventual disappearance of the primitive carotid-basilar anastomoses.

Most of these changes are complete and in the adult configuration by 8 weeks of gestation. For a review and further details, see Osborn's detailed descriptions.[2] Further details have been described by Larsen[3] and Lasjaunias and colleagues.[4]

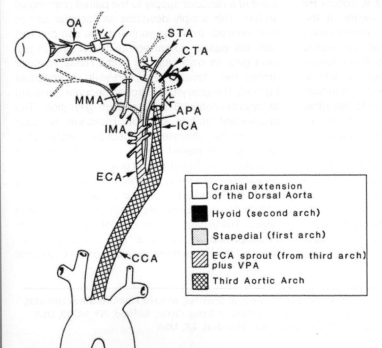

Fig. 1. Anatomic diagram turned from anteroposterior to a left ante-rior oblique position depicts the definitive left common carotid artery (CCA) and the external carotid artery (ECA) and internal carotid artery (ICA). The embryonic origin of these vessels is also shown. Distal ramifications from the internal maxillary artery (IMA), middle meningeal artery (MMA), and orbital branches of the ophthalmic artery (OA) are indicated by the dotted lines. CTA, caroticotympanic artery; STA, stapedial artery; *small single arrow*, stapes; *arrowhead*, foramen spinosum; *double arrows*, optic canal; *open arrows*, carotid canal. (*From* Osborn AG. Diagnostic cere-bral angiography. 2nd edition. Phila-delphia: Lippincott Williams & Wilkins, Wolters Kluwer; 1999; with permission.)

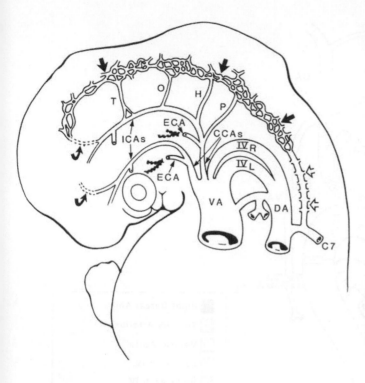

Fig. 2. Three-dimensional sketch at approximately 5 gestational weeks. Development of the paired plexiform longitudinal neural arteries (*solid arrows*). The ventral aortas (VA) (*open arrows*) form as longitudinal anastomoses between the seven cervical intersegmental arteries. The proximal connections between the C1–6 arteries and the dorsal aorta (DA) are regressing. For simplification, only one set of longitudinal neural and cervical intersegmental arteries is shown. These vessels are the precursors of the VB circulation. Initially, the longitudinal neural arteries are supplied from below by the intersegmental arteries. At this stage, several temporary connections between the developing VB circulation and the carotid arteries also form. From cephalad to caudad, these arteries are the trigeminal (T), otic (O), hypoglossal (H), and proatlantal intersegmental arteries (P) (this vessel forms slightly later). These transient anastomoses regress as the caudal divisions of the primitive internal carotid arteries (ICAs) anastomose with the cranial ends of the longitudinal neural arteries and form the future posterior communicating arteries (*dotted lines with curved arrows*). Persistence of the transient embryonic interconnections is abnormal and results in a so-called "primitive carotid–basilar anastomosis." Sprouting of the external carotid arteries (ECAs) from the proximal common carotid arteries (CCAs) is also depicted. These vessels annex first and second arch remnants (*solid black areas*). (*From Osborn AG. Diagnostic cerebral angiography. 2nd edition. Philadelphia: Lippincott Williams & Wilkins, Wolters Kluwer; 1999.*)

EXTRACRANIAL-TO-INTRACRANIAL ANASTOMOSES

For the purpose of grouping these anastomoses, Lasjaunias and colleagues[4,5] and Berenstein and colleagues[6] described regions within the cranial circulation that could be divided on the basis of primitive vascular connections. They divided the regions as follows: (1) anterior or ophthalmic artery connections with facial and internal maxillary arteries; (2) middle or petrocavernous ICA branches with internal maxillary and ascending pharyngeal branches; and (3) posterior or VB connections with ascending pharyngeal, occipital, and subclavian artery branches, especially the ascending and deep cervical arteries.

This division, although overlapping, serves to identify vascular territories of concern (ie, functional areas in which anastomotic dysfunction may become most apparent), thereby tailoring angiographic and neurologic examination during intraprocedural monitoring. Even when not apparent on routine angiography, these connections exist as by-products of a unified vascular

development for the entire head and neck region.[7] Under situations of increased flow, such as with arteriovenous fistulas or arteriovenous malformations, there may be arterioarterial embolization, resulting in deficits. In other cases, shared venous outflow may complicate options or results. Similarly, simply injecting materials, whether contrast or embolic materials, particularly liquid agents, may result in their transfer across the anastomosis to occlude functional vessels supplying neural tissues and result in deficits. In addition, as embolization proceeds and the desired target vessel occludes, putative collateral anastomoses may be at increased risk. This may occur because of their presence as a relative lower-pressure sump (in the face of an occluded principal target vessel), resulting in the preferential shunting of embolic materials into these collaterals.[8] Although these collaterals may increase the risk of embolization procedures in the skull base, they serve to provide critical collaterals in the face of acute or subacute carotid or VB occlusion. They provide an innate bypass that grows under an increased demand

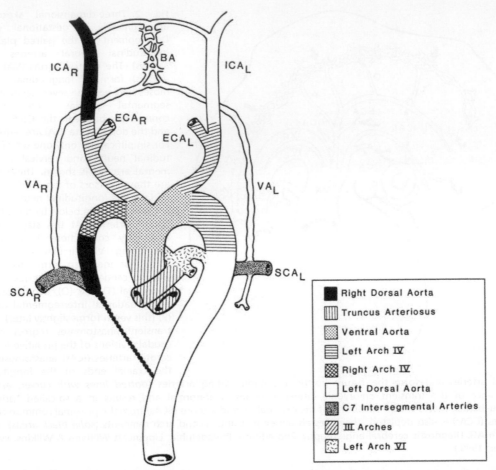

Fig. 3. Diagrammatic sketch of the craniocerebral vasculature at 7 weeks of development. The arch and great vessels are approaching their definitive form. Origins of these vessels from their embryonic precursors are depicted schematically. The fourth and sixth aortic arches are undergoing asymmetric remodeling to supply blood to the upper extremities, dorsal aorta, and lungs. The right sixth arch has involuted (leaving only part of the right pulmonary artery). The right dorsal aorta distal to the origin of the subclavian artery (SCA) is regressing (*dotted lines*) but remains connected to the right fourth arch. The right third and fourth arches are forming the brachiocephalic trunk; the left fourth arch becomes the definitive aortic arch. The left dorsal aorta becomes the proximal descending aorta. The first six cervical intersegmental arteries have become the definitive vertebral arteries (VAs); the C7 arteries have enlarged to become part of the developing subclavian arteries (SCAs). The longitudinal neural arteries are fusing across the midline to form the definitive basilar artery (BA). (*From Osborn AG. Diagnostic cerebral angiography. 2nd edition. Philadelphia: Lippincott Williams & Wilkins, Wolters Kluwer; 1999.*)

from a hypoperfused intracranial territory. A recent review by Geibprasert and colleagues[1] describes these extracranial-intracranial anastomoses in considerable detail. These anastomotic connections are summarized in **Table 1**.

Ophthalmic Artery Anastomoses

The ophthalmic artery is the principal vascular supply for contents in the orbit.[9] It is the principal supply to the central retinal artery, which in turn supplies the retina and choroid. Occlusion of this vessel results in monocular blindness.

Visualization of a choroid blush with an ECA injection should raise alarms about potential anatomic variations and dangerous collaterals.[10] The ophthalmic artery originates from the ICA; however, during its development, it necessarily develops connections with other sources of supply to the contents of the orbit. The primitive stapedial artery contributes to the middle meningeal artery, and this develops some connections to the ophthalmic artery through the superior orbital fissure.[11] The magnitude of this connection may vary; rarely, the middle meningeal and internal maxillary arteries completely assume the principal

Table 1
Extracranial-to-intracranial anastomoses

Location	External Carotid Artery Branch	Internal Carotid Artery Branch
Orbit, superior orbital fissure	Internal maxillary artery: middle meningeal artery	Ophthalmic artery: orbital branches
Falx	Internal maxillary artery: middle meningeal artery	Ophthalmic artery: anterior falcine artery
Orbit	Internal maxillary artery: deep temporal artery, inferior orbital artery	Ophthalmic artery: orbital branches (lacrimal branches)
Ethmoidal sinus	Internal maxillary artery: septal, sphenopalatine, greater palatine arteries	Ophthalmic artery: anterior and posterior ethmoidal arteries
Scalp	Superficial temporal artery	Ophthalmic artery: superior orbital artery
Nose	Facial artery: nasal branches, internal maxillary artery: inferior orbital artery	Ophthalmic artery: dorsal nasal artery
Cavernous sinus	Internal maxillary artery: middle meningeal artery, accessory meningeal artery, deep temporal artery, artery of the foramen rotundum	Internal carotid artery: inferolateral trunk
Sphenopalatine fossa	Internal maxillary artery: artery of the vidian canal	Internal carotid artery: branch of the foramen lacerum (primitive stapedial artery)
Inferotemporal fossa	Internal maxillary artery: accessory meningeal artery	Internal carotid artery: inferolateral trunk (artery of the foramen ovale)
Superior nasopharynx	Ascending pharyngeal artery: pharyngeal branches	Internal carotid artery: artery of the foramen lacerum
Petrous bone: middle ear	Ascending pharyngeal branches: neuromeningeal branches	Internal carotid artery: caroticotympanic branch
Hypoglossal canal and jugular foramen	Ascending pharyngeal branches: neuromeningeal branches (hypoglossal canal and jugular foramen branches)	Internal carotid artery: meningohypophyseal trunk
Odontoid process	Ascending pharyngeal artery: neuromeningeal branches	Vertebral artery: odontoid arch
Stylomastoid foramen	Posterior auricular, occipital artery: stylomastoid branch	Internal carotid artery: caroticotympanic branch (facial nerve supply)
Transverse process of C1	Occipital artery: muscular branches	Vertebral artery: muscular branches
Posterior cervical muscles/fascia	Deep and ascending cervical arteries: muscular branches	Vertebral artery: muscular branches

source of supply to the ophthalmic artery. In cases in which the ophthalmic artery is not visualized, such variation should be suspected.

The anastomotic connections of the ECA branches with the ophthalmic artery may be divided according to the segments of the ophthalmic artery.[9] The first segment of the ophthalmic artery arises as the first supraclinoidal branch of the ICA and travels on the underside of the optic nerve in the optic canal. On entering the orbit, it maintains its close relationship with the optic nerve traveling toward the posterior globe. The recurrent meningeal artery is a reliable branch often noted by microvascular surgeons along the lateral aspect of the superior orbital fissure and is a branch of the middle meningeal artery. This supplies the contents of the superior orbital fissure and then anastomoses with the second segment of the ophthalmic artery in the orbit. This anastomosis is of particular importance when embolizing the middle meningeal artery branches, particularly for convexity meningiomas. The recurrent meningeal artery can often be visualized as the middle meningeal artery crosses the sphenoid wing. In cases in which embolization is desirable, it is best to obtain distal access close to or in the tumor proper and be vigilant to reflux to this more proximal branch point. In other cases in which such a branch is not noted, an intra-arterial injection of sodium amytal and lidocaine may allow Wada testing[12] of the anastomosis, which may not be apparent (**Figs. 4** and **5**).

The second group of anastomoses is a product of the shared supply to the ethmoidal sinuses from the anterior and posterior branches of the ophthalmic artery and branches from septal, sphenopalatine, and greater palatine branches of the internal maxillary artery.[13] These occur along the second and third segments of the ophthalmic artery. In addition, anastomoses may also exist between the

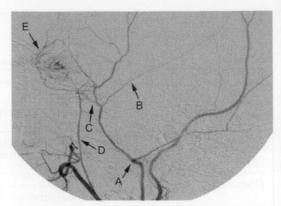

Fig. 5. Selective ECA angiogram reveals a tumor blush of an anterior cranial fossa meningioma. The principal supply is the middle meningeal artery (A), which divides into the parietal branch (B) and an enlarged recurrent meningeal branch (C) that, along with the accessory meningeal artery (D), is the principal supply for this tumor (E, tumor blush).

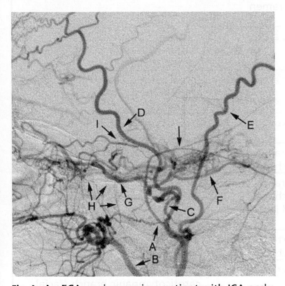

Fig. 4. An ECA angiogram in a patient with ICA occlusion, with reconstitution of the ICA through collaterals by the ophthalmic artery and the cavernous ICA. The vidian artery (A) is supplying collateral flow from the internal maxillary artery (B) to the petrous ICA (C). The frontal branch of the superficial temporal artery (D) is providing transosseous collaterals to the frontal meningo-pial collaterals, whereas the parietal branch (E) is not involved. The PCoA (F) is involved in the extensive neovascularization through its perforators, typical of moyamoya disease. The ophthalmic artery (G) is the largest source of retrograde collateral flow to the ICA. It is receiving its supply principally through its ethmoidal arteries (H) by connections with the internal maxillary artery. Another source of supply to the ophthalmic artery is the recurrent meningeal branch (I) of the middle meningeal artery.

ophthalmic artery and deep temporal and infraorbital branches of the internal maxillary artery. These arise particularly because of shared ophthalmic and internal maxillary supply to the lacrimal apparatus (see **Fig. 4**). These anastomotic connections carry great significance during embolization for epistaxis. Most of the anastomotic connections through the lacrimal and ethmoidal arteries tend to be very small-caliber vessels (less than 80 μm). If embolization is desired, particles chosen should be greater than 150 μm. This prevents inadvertent passage of these particles into the ICA or ophthalmic artery through these collaterals. One needs to identify an aberrant ophthalmic artery origin by always performing a cerebral angiogram to identify the origin of the ophthalmic artery from the ICA. Embolization of anterior fossa-based tumors, such as olfactory groove meningiomas, is considered high risk because the principal supply to these tumors is from the ethmoidal arteries, and transinternal maxillary or transophthalmic embolization of these branches may have an inordinate increased risk for some of the material refluxing into the central retinal artery or retrograde into the ICA (see **Fig. 5**).[13] Another consideration is with falcine meningiomas in which the anterior falcine artery, a branch of the ophthalmic artery, may anastomose with frontal branches of the middle meningeal artery, with retrograde flux of embolization materials into the ophthalmic artery from a middle meningeal artery branch embolization. Other situations in which these anastomoses need to be considered are during embolization for tumors in the head and neck region, particularly juvenile angiofibromas. Cavernous sinus dural arteriovenous fistulas are particularly challenging because their inherent incorporation of these varied collateral channels may create significant risk for transarterial embolization (**Fig. 6**).

The third group of anastomoses occurs along the third or terminal segments of the ophthalmic artery and its terminal branches, the dorsal nasal artery and superior orbital artery (**Fig. 7**). The superior orbital artery anastomoses with the frontal branches of the superficial temporal artery. This anastomosis may gain relevance in situations in which the ICA is occluded with connections by the superior orbital artery supplying the ophthalmic artery and, in some cases, direct transosseous collaterals to frontal cortical meningopial anastomoses (see **Fig. 4**). The dorsal nasal artery anastomoses with terminal nasal branches of the facial artery and the inferior orbital artery (a terminal branch of the internal maxillary artery) (see **Fig. 7**). These anastomoses, particularly the latter, are of great significance during embolization procedures for epistaxis. A high-pressure

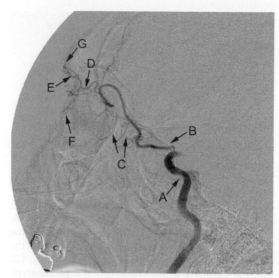

Fig. 7. Selective ICA injection demonstrates an occlusion beyond the origin of the ophthalmic artery. The ICA (A) gives rise to the ophthalmic artery (B), which is its first supraclinoidal branch. The ophthalmic artery then gives rise to multiple ethmoidal arteries (C), terminating as the dorsal nasal artery (D) and the supraorbital artery (E), which passes through the supraorbital notch (G) to anastomose with branches from the frontal branch of the superficial temporal artery. Inferiorly, the dorsal nasal artery anastomoses with the terminal angular branch of the facial artery (F).

angiogram through the microcatheter (microangiogram) before embolization may allow better identification of such dangerous collaterals as compared with an ECA angiogram from a more proximal location.

Petrocavernous Internal Carotid Artery Collaterals

The anastomoses that fall within this region are complex and prone to multiple variations. Only the principal trunks are seen in good-quality angiograms. Although always there, these collateral pathways only become apparent in cases of increased flow across these connections, such as during petrocavernous arteriovenous fistula embolization or after cervical ICA occlusion (see **Figs. 4** and **6; Fig. 8**). A systematic discussion has recently been provided in detail by Geibprasert and colleagues.[1] To understand the organization of these collaterals, one can look at these putative connections in terms of branches of the ICA, which are involved in the anastomosis. The first branch traveling rostrocaudal or distal to proximal along the ICA is the inferolateral trunk off the ICA in the cavernous sinus.

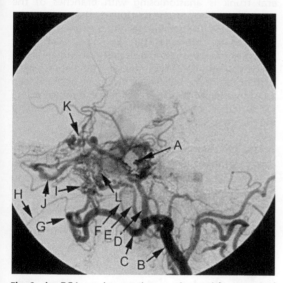

Fig. 6. An ECA angiogram in a patient with a surgical ICA occlusion and cavernous dural arteriovenous fistulas (DAVF) caused by a gun shot (A). The hypertrophied ECA trunk (B) is supplying an enlarged internal maxillary artery (C) and its principal branches: middle meningeal artery (D), accessory meningeal artery (E), deep temporal artery (F), and sphenopalatine artery (G). The sphenopalatine artery branches to supply the small infraorbital artery (H), and the numerous septal arteries communicate with the ethmoidal arteries (I) to supply the enlarged ophthalmic artery (J). The enlarged recurrent meningeal branch (K) is noted off the middle meningeal artery. The accessory meningeal artery is seen communicating with the inferolateral trunk and artery of the foramen rotundum (L), with its typical corkscrew shape.

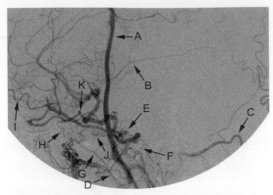

Fig. 8. An ECA angiogram following successful bypass with a radial artery graft from the ECA to the MCA. The radial artery graft (A) can be seen overlaid on the cavernous sinus anastomosis. Parietal branch of the middle meningeal artery (B). Occipital artery (C). Internal maxillary artery trunk (D). The caroticotympanic artery (E) anastomoses with branches from the ascending pharyngeal branches (F) to reconstitute the ICA. The accessory meningeal artery (G) is anastomosing with the inferolateral trunk branches. Additionally, the ethmoidal vessels (H) are supplying the ophthalmic artery (K). The inferolateral trunk is anastomosing with branches from the middle meningeal branches at the foramen spinosum (J) and through the artery of the foramen rotundum more anteriorly.

The inferolateral trunk has multiple branches, which supply the anterior and middle parts of the cavernous sinus structures.[4,14–16] It is a remnant of an embryologic dorsal ophthalmic artery and connects to its ECA counterparts principally along the foramina of cranial nerves or in the meningeal walls of the cavernous sinus. Anteriorly, it communicates with the internal maxillary artery through the artery of the foramen rotundum; laterally, it collateralizes with the cavernous branches of the middle meningeal artery, which arise soon after the artery exits the foramen spinosum; and, posteriorly, it communicates with the accessory meningeal artery through the artery of foramen ovale (see **Fig. 8**).

The second branch in this order is a remnant of the primitive stapedial artery and the subsequent mandibular trunk off the stapediohyoid artery, a small branch that pierces the foramen lacerum arising either directly off the carotid artery or as a branch off the meningohypophyseal trunk, which enters the vidian canal to anastomose with the sphenopalatine artery (a branch of the internal maxillary artery in the sphenopalatine fossa).[17] It also anastomoses with the superior pharyngeal artery (a branch of the pharyngeal trunk of the ascending pharyngeal artery) and the accessory meningeal artery to provide a branch to the pterygovaginal canal, which ends by anastomosing with internal maxillary artery branches (**Fig. 9**).

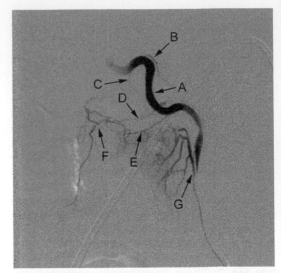

Fig. 9. Selective microinjection in an occluded ICA demonstrating connections with extracranial vessels. The ICA (A) is occluded at the distal cavernous segment. Its cavernous branches, the meningohypophyseal trunk (B) and inferolateral trunk (C), are noted. The inferolateral trunk is anastomosing with branches of the internal maxillary artery, particularly the sphenopalatine artery (F), through the artery of the foramen rotundum. More inferiorly, the primitive mandibular (petrous) branch anastomoses with the vidian artery (D), which originates from the sphenopalatine artery. Further inferiorly, the caroticotympanic artery is seen anastomosing with the ascending pharyngeal artery (G); together, these vessels are supplying the artery of the pterygovaginal canal (E).

The third branch of note is the primitive maxillary artery remnant, the meningohypophyseal trunk. This branch has widespread connections along the posterior cavernous sinus and clivus. Anteriorly, it anastomoses through its tentorial branch

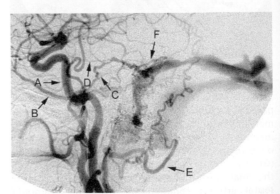

Fig. 10. A CCA angiogram revealing a transverse-sigmoid junction DAVF. ICA (A). The middle meningeal artery's (B) petrous branch (C) is supplying the DAVF, as is the tentorial branch (D) of the meningohypophyseal trunk of the ICA. The transosseous branches from the occipital artery (E) are a major supply to the DAVF (F).

(of Bernasconi and Cassinari) with petrous branches from the middle meningeal artery. These branches are particularly noted during angiography for superior petrosal sinus or transverse-sigmoid junction dural arteriovenous fistulas (**Fig. 10**). More posteriorly, its major branch, the lateral clival artery, anastomoses extensively with neuromeningeal branches of the ascending pharyngeal artery, including branches that supply the hypoglossal and jugular foramina.

The most proximal branch of the ICA is the caroticotympanic artery in the petrous canal.[16,18–20] This embryologic remnant of the hyoid artery anastomoses with the tympanic plexus, which is supplied by the tympanic branches of the ascending pharyngeal artery, stylomastoid artery from the posterior auricular artery, and petrotympanic branches of the middle meningeal artery (see **Fig. 9**).

These branches become most apparent as vascular sources for cavernous and petroclival meningiomas or for tympanic or jugular foramen glomus tumors. Because of the critical supply to cranial nerves and their ganglia in these foramina, embolization of these vessels carries potential for lower cranial nerve dysfunction.

Vertebrobasilar Anastomoses

The VB system develops through posterior paired longitudinal arteries that coalesce rostrally to form the basilar artery, whereas inferiorly they remain separate as VAs. Rostrally, this system is supplied through collaterals of which only the PCoA remains in most adults. Primitive anastomoses include the trigeminal artery, which remains as a branch to Meckel's cave; the otic artery, as the labyrinthine artery; the hypoglossal artery, as an artery to the hypoglossal canal; and the proatlantal artery, as the occipital artery and its connections

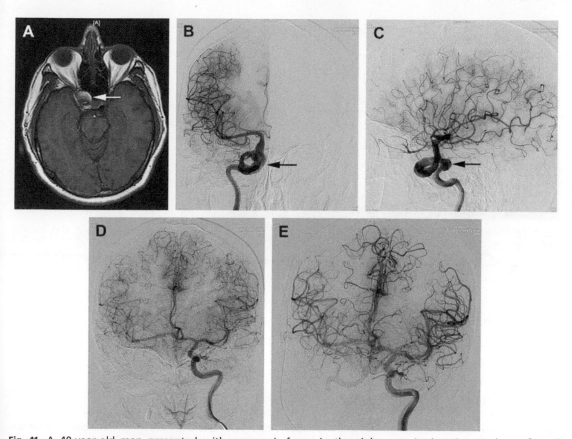

Fig. 11. A 40-year-old man presented with amaurosis fugax in the right eye. An imaging study confirmed a partially thrombosed giant aneurysm of the right ICA cavernous segment that likely had caused the embolic event. (*A*) T1-weighted MRI reveals a partially thrombosed cavernous aneurysm (*arrow*). (*B, C*) Angiography shows the fusiform aneurysm with serpentine channel (*arrow*). (*D*) Right ICA temporary balloon occlusion (TBO) test with angiogram from left ICA reveals robust cross-filling of the contralateral circulation. The anterior communicating artery (ACoA) serves to opacify the right ACA and MCA without delay. (*E*) The patient tolerated TBO and was successfully treated with right ICA sacrifice.

to the VA over the first cervical vertebra and separately at the second cervical vertebra, through segmental vertebral branches. Although regressed, these connections may remain viable and become prominent under conditions of increased flow. Rarely, they remain as principal supply to the posterior circulation with regression of the more proximal VB system.[21–23]

The occipital artery routinely has a prominent connection to the VA as it emerges from the C1 transverse foramen. Embolization of dural arteriovenous fistulas, particularly those involving the transverse sinuses at the transverse sigmoid junction or torcula, can have enlarged occipital feeders; care must be exercised to ensure that no inadvertent posterior circulation embolization occurs. In other situations, this route may be used to treat intracranial lesions, such as acute occlusions,[24] or other pathologic conditions.

The neuromeningeal trunk of the ascending pharyngeal artery anastomoses with the VA

through connections at C3 through muscular collaterals and, more rostrally, as the remnant of the primitive hypoglossal artery with the odontoid arch vascular system.[25,26]

More caudally, the cervical branches of the subclavian artery anastomose with proximal sections of the VAs (C3–7). The ascending cervical artery arises from the thyrocervical trunk, whereas the deep cervical artery arises from the costocervical trunk. Both these branches form connections with the segmental vertebral branches through muscular collaterals. They are commonly noted to reconstitute the distal VA after proximal occlusion.

Complication Avoidance

First and foremost, one needs to be aware of the potential for collateral anastomotic channels. Such knowledge facilitates angiographic visualization. Even if the initial proximal external carotid or

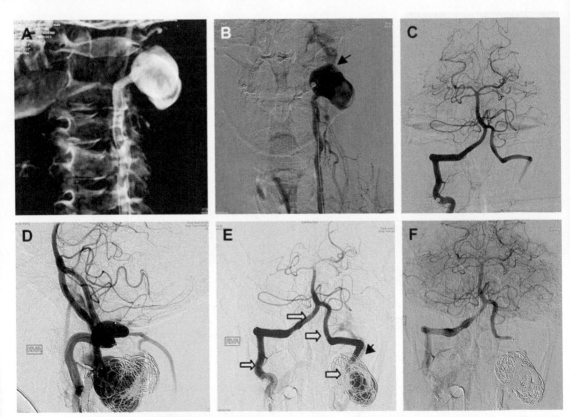

Fig. 12. A 38-year-old man with a left PCA territory embolic infarct was found to have a traumatic giant left VA dissecting aneurysm and DAVF from a fall 2 years before treatment. (*A, B*) Three-dimensional and two-dimensional angiograms show a giant left VA dissecting aneurysm and a DAVF. (*C*) The right VA angiogram demonstrates competent flow in the right VA. (*D, E*) Because of extremely high flow in the giant aneurysm, the DAVF was unable to be catheterized until occlusion of the left VA at the origin of the aneurysm. The left traumatic vertebral DAVF was catheterized from the right VA through the VB junction to the left VA (fistula, *black arrowhead*; microcatheter route, *open arrows*). (*F*) The fistula and residual filling of the giant aneurysm were treated successfully with coil occlusion through the contralateral VA to the left vertebral DAVF and giant aneurysm.

subclavian angiograms do not result in the visualization of these collaterals, it is recommended that selective microcatheter angiograms be performed in as distal a position as is reasonably attainable immediately before embolization. These higher pressure selective injections are more likely to reveal these putative connections. If there is no visualization, a second element to bolster confidence further is to perform a Wada test with sodium amytal (75 mg) and lidocaine (30 mg) intra-arterially through the microcatheter from the position planned for embolization and then immediately after injection to test for loss of appropriate neural function including that of the cranial nerves. Thirdly, if embolization is desired, polyvinyl alcohol particles, which considerably exceed the size (150 μm or greater) of most of these non-angiographically

visualized collaterals (50–80 μm), should be used. Liquid embolics, such as glue (N-butyl cyanoacrylate; Trufill, Codman Neurovascular, Raynham, Massachusetts) and Onyx (ev3, Irvine, California), provide superior visualization; however, they are not discriminatory with respect to vessel size and their use may be associated with a higher likelihood of collateral vessel occlusion.

Angiographic visualization does not preclude embolization. One may attempt to attain distal purchase beyond the collateral communication and pay great attention to reflux during the embolization procedure. If such positioning is not attainable, pre-embolization occlusion of the collateral channel is another strategy. Typically, coil embolization of the collateral channel does not result in ischemic injury because of the multiple sources of

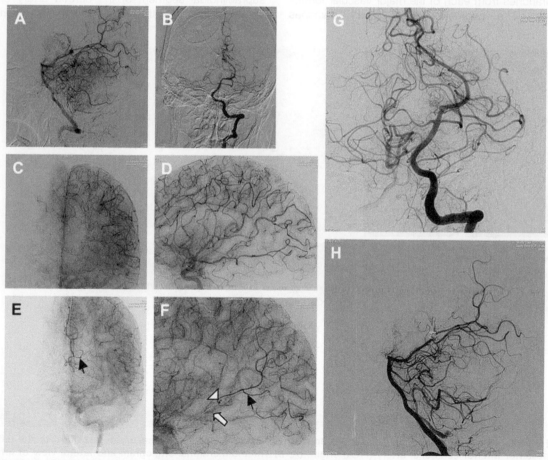

Fig. 13. A 48-year-old woman with a subarachnoid hemorrhage caused by a left P2–P3 junction ruptured aneurysm. (*A, B*) Lateral view and anteroposterior (AP) view of original VA angiogram. (*C, D*) Left ICA AP and lateral angiography. (*E, F*) Left PCA P2 TBO. The left ICA angiogram, while the left P2 was occluded with a balloon, revealed left ACA to PCA cortical collateralization (*black arrowhead*) with retrograde opacification during the late arterial phase. In *F, open arrow* indicates the balloon; *arrowhead* indicates the retrograde partially opacified P2-P3 aneurysm. (*G, H*) Ultimately, this aneurysm was coil embolized completely with balloon-remodeling technique, and the distal PCA branches were preserved anterograde.

vascular supply at the skull base; however, subsequent embolization of the intended vessel prevents inadvertent passage of embolic materials through the occluded vessel to critical neural structures.

INTRACRANIAL ANASTOMOSES

In contrast to the extracranial-to-intracranial collateral anastomoses described previously, which may be less obvious on nonsuperselective angiography, many of the ICA-to-ICA or ICA-to-VB anastomoses are rather easily identified and commonly seen. These commonly known collateral anastomoses as parts of the circle of Willis include the following: anterior communicating artery connecting bilateral anterior cerebral arteries (ACAs); and PCoA connecting the ipsilateral ICA to the posterior cerebral artery (PCA). Less obvious anastomoses occur among the various terminal cortical branches from each of the major vascular territories. The middle cerebral artery branches

anastomose with branches of the PCA and ACA. The pericallosal branches of the ACA connect to splenial branches of PCA. Distal branches of the superior cerebellar artery connect to branches from posterior inferior cerebellar artery. These anastomoses not only provide collaterals to preserve potentially affected brain tissue in the case of an occlusion event, but also provide crucial collateral supply if carotid artery or VA sacrifice becomes necessary; also, potentially, the collaterals may be used as alternative access routes to the target during interventional procedures.

Intracranial Collateralization in Neurointerventional Procedures

Flow replacement by collateral vessels
Intracranial large artery sacrifice In patients with fusiform or giant aneurysms of the cavernous or supraclinoidal segment of the carotid artery or supraclinoidal carotid artery dissection with

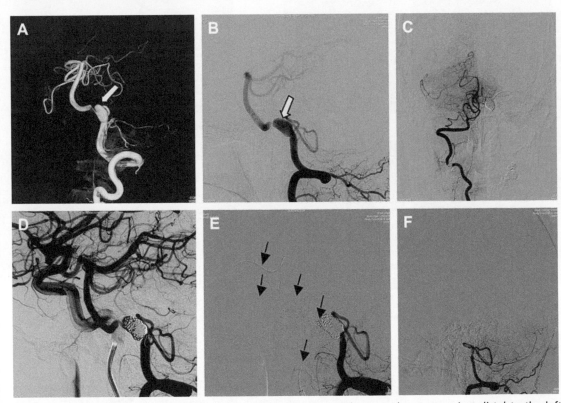

Fig. 14. A 40-year-old man with a left intracranial VA dissection with a pseudoaneurysm just distal to the left posterior inferior cerebellar artery (PICA) origin. (*A, B*) Three-dimensional angiogram and lateral view of left VA two-dimensional angiogram (pseudoaneurysm at the dissection site, *arrows*). (*C*) Left ICA angiogram revealed robust PCoA connecting the left ICA system to the VB system. (*D*) Because of limited distal flow from the dissecting aneurysm to the normal PICA origin, complete occlusion of the left VA was not achieved by balloon-remodeling coiling through left VA catheterization. Superselective catheterization through a left ICA–PCoA–BA–left VA route allowed successful occluding of the diseased segment of the VA. *Arrows* in *E* indicate the microcatheter route. By comparison with the angiogram in *C*, the 3-month follow-up angiogram with right VA (*E*) and left VA (*F,* lateral view) runs shows the left VA supplying the left PICA without evidence of recurrent aneurysm.

hemorrhage, sacrifice of the ipsilateral ICA can be a simple therapeutic solution with low risk if the anterior communicating artery and PCoA provide sufficient cross-filling to the affected side. This is especially true if both angiographic and neurophysiologic tests are completed during a temporary balloon occlusion test (**Fig. 11**).[27–29] It should be noted that endovascular strategies for

vessel preservation during treatment continue gradually to erode options for vessel sacrifice.

Sacrifice of the VA is an effective strategy for the management of pathologic conditions of the VA, such as dissection with hemorrhage or endovascularly unmanageable aneurysms, simply because most patients are endowed with two vessels; after the sacrifice of one, unabated flow typically

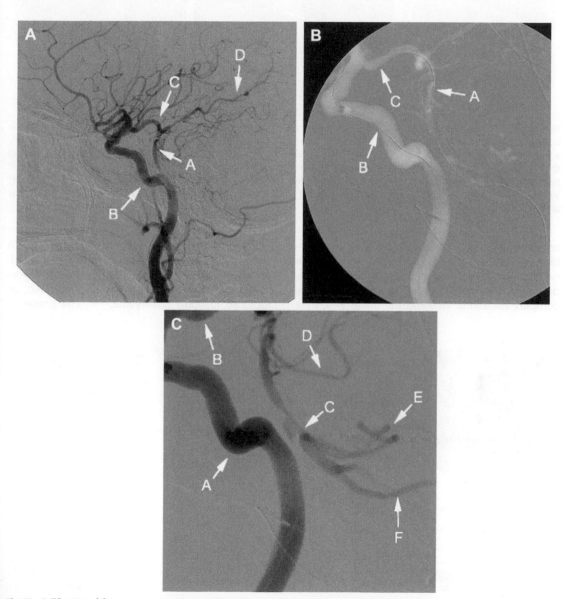

Fig. 15. A 70-year-old woman presented with multiple events of VB insufficiency. Evaluation revealed bilateral VA occlusions. (*A*) Injection of the left ICA (C) revealed the PCoA (B) as the principal supply to the BA (A) and the PCA (D). (*B*) A road-map angiogram reveals a guide catheter in the left ICA (B) with a microwire through the PCoA (C) and through the proximal BA (A) across an obvious stenosis into the distal VA. (*C*) After retrograde BA angioplasty, an ICA (A) angiogram reveals robust filling through the PCoA (B) into the basilar artery with markedly improved flow across the stenotic lesion into the BA junction (C), bilateral PICA, and VA (E, F). (*From* Chiam PT, Mocco J, Samuelson RM, et al. Retrograde angioplasty for basilar artery stenosis: bypassing bilateral vertebral artery occlusions. J Neurosurg 2009;110:427–30.)

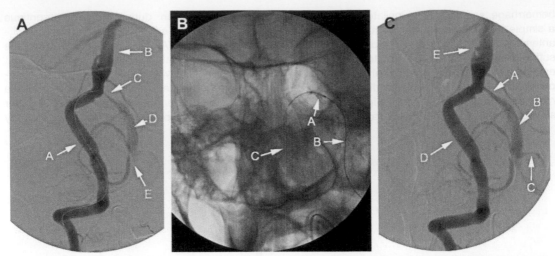

Fig. 16. A 65-year-old man presented with neck movement–related VB insufficiency. The left VA was noted to be occluded extracranially. (*A*) Right VA (A) angiogram revealed excellent flow into the BA with fenestration (B), a tight stenosis at the junction (C) of the left VA (D) with the BA, and a peak systolic angiographic jet opacifying the PICA (E). (*B*) A microballoon (A) was brought from the right VA (C) over a wire, which was placed into the left proximal VA (B). (*C*) Final angiogram revealing significant improvement (despite persistent stenosis) in distal left VA (A) flow noted into the proximal left VA (B) and left PICA (C) following a right VA (D) injection. (E) Basilar artery.

continues through the other. It is, however, important that the temporary balloon occlusion test be performed before a vessel deconstruction procedure is performed (**Fig. 12**). There are other more complex situations involving the distal VAs, their junction, or the basilar artery in which neither VA can be preserved nor flow reversal is desired. These situations include dissections with hemorrhage and complex, enlarging, symptomatic, or ruptured fusiform aneurysms.[30,31] The presence

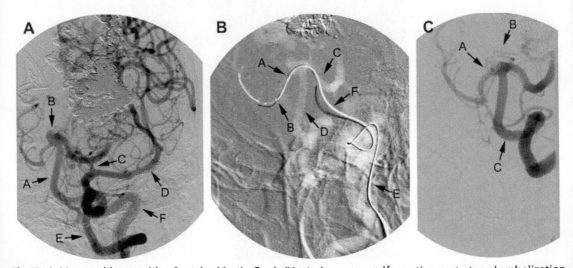

Fig. 17. A 44-year-old man with a Spetzler-Martin Grade IV arteriovenous malformation post–staged embolization and Gamma Knife radiosurgery presented with a residual, broad-based basilar terminus aneurysm. (*A*) Combined left carotid (E) and left VA (F) angiogram reveals a robust PCoA (C). BA (A), aneurysm (B), MCA (D). (*B*) Road-map image of an Enterprise stent (Codman Neurovascular, Raynham, Massachusetts) being deployed by the left ICA (E) through the left PCoA (F) from the ipsilateral P1 segment of the PCA (C) across the neck of the aneurysm into the contralateral PCA (B). Deployed stent markers (A). BA (D). (*C*) The patient was subsequently brought for a second coil embolization session with access to the BA aneurysm achieved from the left VA (C). Angiographically, complete aneurysm obliteration (A) was obtained. The left PCoA (B) is noted.

of a robust PCoA and a large-caliber ipsilateral PCA P1 segment may allow sacrifice of both VAs, thereby creating flow reversal with a diminution of flow, enough to reduce hemodynamic stresses on the diseased vessel and allowing it to heal. It should be borne in mind that, before such deconstruction, which is undoubtedly high risk, a comprehensive angiographic evaluation including a VA angiogram with transient bilateral manual carotid artery compression can be very useful to identify bilateral PCoA. Further hemodynamic and neurophysiologic testing should be completed before vessel deconstruction.

Intracranial distal end-artery sacrifice Occasionally, one may encounter dissecting, mycotic, or ruptured broad-based aneurysms involving the distal ACA, middle cerebral artery, or PCA and considered high risk for surgical or endovascular reconstruction. Because of well-developed cortical collaterals from ipsilateral ACA to PCA or middle cerebral artery to PCA or ACA to middle cerebral artery territories, these collaterals typically are revealed or opacified during angiography only after proximal vessel test occlusion. The authors typically perform a microballoon test occlusion of the proximal vessel (as distal as possible remaining proximal to the aneurysm). Under microvessel occlusion, they perform proximal angiograms and concurrent neurophysiologic testing to demonstrate angiographic and functional collateralization. If the patient tolerates the test occlusion, they then proceed immediately with endovascular embolization and permanent occlusion of the tested vessel distal to the test site (**Fig. 13**). If the patient does not tolerate test

occlusion, one then has to weigh the risks of vessel-preserving strategies through microsurgical or endovascular means versus the expected neurologic deficit of vessel deconstruction. It should be noted that Hallacq and colleagues[32] reported a series of 10 cases of P2 PCA aneurysms treated with occlusion of the aneurysm and parent vessel without balloon test occlusion in which no postocclusion occipital lobe ischemia occurred.

Alternative microcatheterization of target vessel by a collateral route
The circle of Willis provides a natural conduit to access contralateral or carotid to basilar (or vice versa) circulations. In most cases, adequate access may be obtained through direct ipsilateral routes; however, because of either proximal vessel occlusion or distal vessel entry angles, these alternate routes through the circle of Willis provide easier microcatheter entry angles.

A sharp reversely angulated origin of a vessel makes superselective ipsilateral catheterization difficult. For instance, access to the posterior inferior cerebellar artery or anterior inferior cerebellar artery from the VA can be occasionally difficult, or in cases in which the carotid or bilateral VAs are occluded, the PCoA offers a distinct advantage. In these situations, if the caliber of the PCoA is adequate, effective catheterization of the desired vessel can be achieved (**Figs. 14** and **15**). Naturally, a microcatheter can also go from one VA to the other through the VB junction (see **Fig. 12; Fig. 16**).[33] Similarly, during treatment of broad-based aneurysms at the basilar or ICA terminus, ipsilateral placement of a stent may be

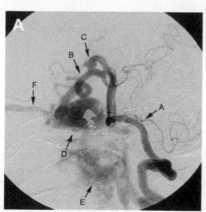 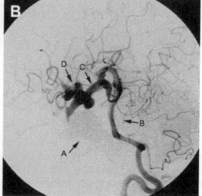

Fig. 18. A 40-year-old man presented with a history of a bullet injury to the head and neck and surgical ligation of the left ICA and now with acute development of a carotid-cavernous fistula. He was noted to have a ruptured, giant, cavernous ICA pseudoaneurysm. (*A*) A left VA (A) angiogram reveals filling of the aneurysm (D) across the PCoA (C) to the supraclinoidal carotid artery (B) with early venous filling of the ophthalmic vein (F) and pterygoid venous plexus (E). (*B*) The aneurysm was accessed through the same route from the left VA (B) across the PCoA (C) to achieve complete obliteration of the aneurysm and carotid-cavernous fistula (A). MCA (D).

inadequate for complete coverage of the aneurysm neck, necessitating a Y-configuration with increased risk of thromboembolic complications. In these cases, the following strategies offer distinct advantages: access from the contralateral carotid artery to pass a stent across the anterior communicating artery so that it ultimately sits across the entire neck of the aneurysm in the ICA terminus (from the ipsilateral ACA to the middle cerebral artery); or access from the carotid artery across the PCoA so that it sits from the ipsilateral

PCA to contralateral PCA (**Fig. 17**). In cases in which there is occlusion of one or more vessels to the circle of Willis, the circle provides an optimal opportunity to access diseased segments of vessels that are proximally occluded. These routes can be used to treat a variety of conditions, such as aneurysms (**Fig. 18**), arteriovenous malformations, or arteriovenous fistulas. Similarly, in cases of acute occlusion, even if the proximal vessel cannot be adequately revascularized, re-establishing flow across the circle may alleviate acute

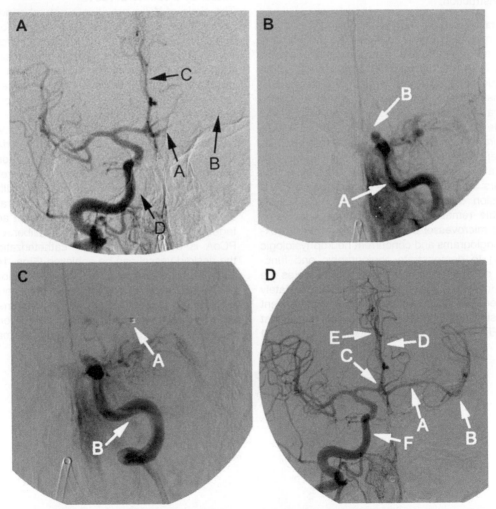

Fig. 19. A 65-year-old man presented with an acute stroke with occlusion of his left ICA. He was beyond the window for intravenous thrombolysis. His ancillary studies suggested potentially viable brain in the MCA territory. CT angiography suggested occlusion of the left MCA territory, however, in addition to more proximal carotid occlusion. An emergent angiogram was planned. (*A*) A right carotid (D) angiogram performed to assess crossflow reveals a left ICA terminus occlusion (A) with flow to the bilateral distal ACA circulation across the ACoA (C) but no flow to the left MCA (B). (*B*) Selective left ICA angiogram reveals complete cavernous occlusion (B) of the left ICA (A). (*C*) The occlusion (B) was carefully crossed, and a thrombectomy suction catheter (A) was advanced into the occluded left MCA. (*D*) Following suction aspiration, the clot was retrieved from the MCA (B), resulting in revascularization of the ICA terminus (A) and re-establishment of flow across the ACoA (C) from the right ICA (F). Both ACAs remained patent (E, D). Despite these efforts, the proximal occlusion remained recalcitrant to revascularization efforts and was left occluded. The patient recovered from all deficits.

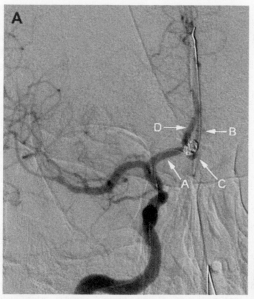 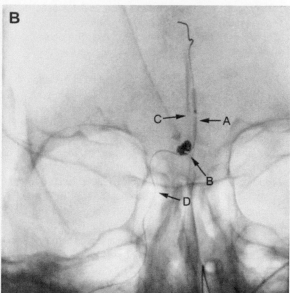

Fig. 20. A 42-year-old man presented with a ruptured ACoA aneurysm, which was treated by coil embolization. On Day 6, he developed severe symptomatic spasm, which remained refractory to maximal medical therapy. He had severe spasm of his left ACA, which resulted in the use of the ACoA artery as a conduit to angioplasty the left distal ACA. (*A*) Right carotid angiogram reveals a microcatheter and wire across the right ACA (A), AcoA, and aneurysm (C) into the left distal ACA (B). Right distal ACA (D). (*B*) Nonsubtracted angiogram revealing the relationship of the aneurysm and the inflated balloon in the left distal ACA (A). AcoA (B), right distal ACA (C). Access microcatheter in the right ICA (D).

cerebral ischemia (**Fig. 19**). In other situations, the circle may allow passage of endovascular implements that, despite patency, cannot be brought up through ipsilateral routes. This is particularly relevant to situations in which the ipsilateral vessel may have spasm after subarachnoid hemorrhage (**Fig. 20**) or be congenitally hypoplastic.

SUMMARY

An in-depth knowledge of intracranial and extracranial collateral anastomoses, overt or hidden, is crucial for an interventionist to devise optimal endovascular strategies to manage a host of pathologic conditions; to ascertain potential pitfalls; and, ultimately, to avoid complications that could have been prevented by a better understanding of underlying vascular anatomy. As the scope and extent of endovascular interventions for cerebrovascular and cranial disease continue to expand, the recognition of these putative anastomoses will continue to become a larger part of diagnostic evaluation and interventional design.

REFERENCES

1. Geibprasert S, Pongpech S, Armstrong D, et al. Dangerous extracranial-intracranial anastomoses and supply to the cranial nerves: vessels the neurointerventionalist needs to know. AJNR Am J Neuroradiol March 11, 2009;doi:10.3174/ajnr.A1500.

2. Osborn AG. Diagnostic cerebral angiography. 2nd edition. Philadelphia: Lippincott Williams & Wilkins, Wolters Kluwer; 1999.

3. Larsen WJ. Development of vasculature. New York: Churchill Livingstone; 1997.

4. Lasjaunias P, Berenstein A, ter Brugge K. Surgical neuroangiography. 1. Clinical vascular anatomy and variations. Berlin: Springer-Verlag; 2001.

5. Lasjaunias P, Berenstein A, ter Brugge K. Surgical neuroangiography. 2. Clinical and endovascular treatment aspects in adults. Berlin: Springer-Verlag; 2004.

6. Berenstein A, Lasjaunias P, Kricheff II. Functional anatomy of the facial vasculature in pathologic conditions and its therapeutic application. AJNR Am J Neuroradiol 1983;4:149–53.

7. Countee RW, Vijayanathan T. External carotid artery in internal carotid artery occlusion. Angiographic, therapeutic, and prognostic considerations. Stroke 1979;10:450–60.

8. Casasco A, Houdart E, Biondi A, et al. Major complications of percutaneous embolization of skull-base tumors. AJNR Am J Neuroradiol 1999;20:179–81.

9. Hayreh SS. Orbital vascular anatomy. Eye 2006;20: 1130–44.

10. Perrini P, Cardia A, Fraser K, et al. A microsurgical study of the anatomy and course of the ophthalmic

artery and its possibly dangerous anastomoses. J Neurosurg 2007;106:142–50.

11. Silbergleit R, Quint DJ, Mehta BA, et al. The persistent stapedial artery. AJNR Am J Neuroradiol 2000; 21:572–7.

12. Wada J. A new method for determination of the side of cerebral speech dominance: a preliminary report of the intra-carotid injection of sodium amytal in man. Igaku Seibutsugaki 1949;14:221–2.

13. Agid R, Terbrugge K, Rodesch G, et al. Management strategies for anterior cranial fossa (ethmoidal) dural arteriovenous fistulas with an emphasis on endovascular treatment. J Neurosurg 2009;110:79–84.

14. Capo H, Kupersmith MJ, Berenstein A, et al. The clinical importance of the inferolateral trunk of the internal carotid artery. Neurosurgery 1991;28:733–8.

15. Lasjaunias P, Moret J, Mink J. The anatomy of the inferolateral trunk (ILT) of the internal carotid artery. Neuroradiology 1977;13:215–20.

16. Tubbs RS, Hansasuta A, Loukas M, et al. Branches of the petrous and cavernous segments of the internal carotid artery. Clin Anat 2007;20:596–601.

17. Takeuchi M, Kuwayama N, Kubo M, et al. Vidian artery as a collateral channel between the external and occluded internal carotid arteries: case report. Neurol Med Chir (Tokyo) 2005;45:470–1.

18. Hacein-Bey L, Daniels DL, Ulmer JL, et al. The ascending pharyngeal artery: branches, anastomoses, and clinical significance. AJNR Am J Neuroradiol 2002;23:1246–56.

19. Osawa S, Rhoton AL Jr, Tanriover N, et al. Microsurgical anatomy and surgical exposure of the petrous segment of the internal carotid artery. Neurosurgery 2008;63:210–39.

20. Osborn AG. The vidian artery: normal and pathologic anatomy. Radiology 1980;136:373–8.

21. Miyachi S, Negoro M, Sugita K. The occipital-vertebral anastomosis as a collateral pathway: hemodynamic patterns: case report. Surg Neurol 1989;32:350–5.

22. Papon X, Pasco A, Fournier HD, et al. Anastomosis between the internal carotid and vertebral artery in the neck. Surg Radiol Anat 1995;17:335–7.

23. Spetzler RF, Modic M, Bonstelle C. Spontaneous opening of large occipital-vertebral artery

anastomosis during embolization: case report. J Neurosurg 1980;53:849–50.

24. Wang H, Fraser K, Wang D, et al. Successful intra-arterial basilar artery thrombolysis in a patient with bilateral vertebral artery occlusion: technical case report. Neurosurgery 2005;57:E398.

25. Haffajee MR. A contribution by the ascending pharyngeal artery to the arterial supply of the odontoid process of the axis vertebra. Clin Anat 1997;10: 14–8.

26. Nakamura M, Kobayashi S, Yoshida T, et al. Persistent external carotid-vertebrobasilar anastomosis via the hypoglossal canal. Neuroradiology 2000;42: 821–3.

27. Chen PR, Ortiz R, Page JH, et al. Spontaneous systolic blood pressure elevation during temporary balloon occlusion increases the risk of ischemic events after carotid artery occlusion. Neurosurgery 2008;63:256–65.

28. Standard SC, Ahuja A, Guterman LR, et al. Balloon test occlusion of the internal carotid artery with hypotensive challenge. AJNR Am J Neuroradiol 1995;16:1453–8.

29. van Rooij WJ, Sluzewski M, Slob MJ, et al. Predictive value of angiographic testing for tolerance to therapeutic occlusion of the carotid artery. AJNR Am J Neuroradiol 2005;26:175–8.

30. Albuquerque FC, Fiorella DJ, Han PP, et al. Endovascular management of intracranial vertebral artery dissecting aneurysms. Neurosurg Focus 2005;18:E3.

31. O'Shaughnessy BA, Getch CC, Bendok BR, et al. Late morphological progression of a dissecting basilar artery aneurysm after staged bilateral vertebral artery occlusion: case report. Surg Neurol 2005;63:236–43.

32. Hallacq P, Piotin M, Moret J. Endovascular occlusion of the posterior cerebral artery for the treatment of p2 segment aneurysms: retrospective review of a 10-year series. AJNR Am J Neuroradiol 2002;23: 1128–36.

33. Chiam PT, Mocco J, Samuelson RM, et al. Retrograde angioplasty for basilar artery stenosis: bypassing bilateral vertebral artery occlusions. J Neurosurg 2009;110:427–30.

Advanced Imaging Applications for Endovascular Procedures

Lisa M. Tartaglino, MD*, Richard J.T. Gorniak, MD

KEYWORDS

• Aneurysm • Stroke • Imaging • CTA • MRA • Perfusion

ACUTE INFARCTION

Cerebrovascular disease is a common source of mortality, with approximately 150,000 stroke-related deaths in the United States in 2004.[1] The majority of strokes are ischemic, caused by thrombus or embolus occluding or critically narrowing intracranial arteries. Intervention to lyse or mechanically disrupt this clot can be used to establish re-perfusion and halt progression of infarction in appropriately selected patients. Although this has the potential to prevent serious neurologic complications and death, these interventions must be used judiciously to decrease secondary intracranial hemorrhage, which can then lead to death or disability.[2] While intravenous tissue plasminogen activator (TPA) is the mainstay of treatment of ischemic stroke in the first 3 hours after symptom onset, endovascular treatment with intra-arterial thrombolysis or mechanical thrombolysis may be useful in patients who did not respond to intravenous (IV) TPA or who present after the 3-hour window.[3,4] In addition to clinical factors, imaging is vital to exclude absolute contraindications, such as hemorrhage, at presentation, and to evaluate factors that impact the likelihood of success, such as the site of arterial occlusion, the extent of completed infarction, and perfusion abnormalities indicating ischemic tissue at risk for infarction.

The initial goal of imaging patients with a clinical suspicion of acute infarction is to rapidly determine whether there is intracranial hemorrhage or an obvious nonvascular stroke mimic, such as tumor or vascular malformation, which would preclude the use of either IV or intra-arterial thrombolysis.[5] This is typically accomplished with a noncontrast CT of the head, which can be obtained rapidly, has no contraindications, and is widely available. In patients with infarctions that are less than 3 hours old, a noncontrast CT is usually normal. MRI with diffusion would be more sensitive for the detection of infarction (**Fig. 1**),[6] though the screening for non-MRI-compatible implanted devices, longer scan time, and decreased availably relative to CT limit the use of MRI in this time-critical setting.

For patients in which intra-arterial thrombolysis or mechanical disruption is considered, determining the presence of a clot amenable to intervention is also necessary. The most studied situation is a clot in the M1 or M2 segment, which was evaluated in the (PROACT II) trial. This showed that treatment with intra-arterial r-proUK within 6 hours of the onset of acute ischemic stroke caused by middle cerebral artery (MCA) occlusion significantly improved clinical outcome at 90 days.[4] The presence of a proximal MCA or carotid thrombus on CT angiography (CTA) predicts a worse outcome after IV TPA than in patients with distal or occult occlusion.[7] Intra-arterial thrombolysis in vertebrobasilar thrombosis is not well studied.[8] However, given the poor prognosis of patients with basilar artery occlusion,[9]

Division of Neuroradiology, Department of Radiology, Thomas Jefferson University and Hospital, 10th Floor Main Building, 132 South 10th Street, Philadelphia, PA 19107, USA
* Corresponding author.
E-mail address: lisa.tartaglino@jefferson.edu (L.M. Tartaglino).

Neurosurg Clin N Am 20 (2009) 297–313
doi:10.1016/j.nec.2009.01.001
1042-3680/09/$ – see front matter © 2009 Elsevier Inc. All rights reserved.

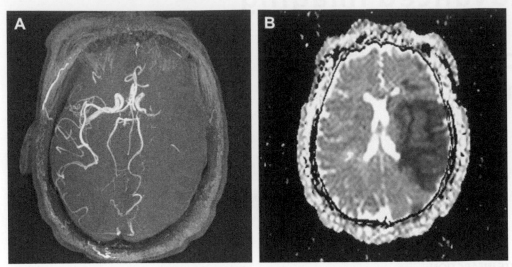

Fig. 1. (A) MR angiography (MRA) showing left middle cerebral artery (LMCA) occlusion. (B) Apparent diffusion coefficient map showing LMCA infarction.

thrombolysis is not uncommonly attempted beyond the timeframe used in the anterior circulation. As an alternative or adjunct, mechanical techniques are also used to disrupt clots in the major intracranial arteries. Mechanical thrombectomy after adjunctive therapy achieved 69.5% recanalization rate in patients with treatable lesions within 8 hours of symptom onset.[3] While the presence of a treatable clot can be determined from a diagnostic cerebral angiogram, similar information can be rapidly obtained noninvasively from CTA. Performing a noninvasive test to determine the presence of a treatable clot first can obviate the need for an invasive digital subtraction angiography (DSA) in cases where no intervention will occur. CTA is typically used in this setting because of its rapid acquisition. Only limited postprocessing of the CTA data is needed in the acute setting, typically multiplanar overlapping thick-slab maximum-intensity projections (MIPs) that can be produced by the CT technologist.[10] These MIP images provide clear depiction of the major intracranial arteries (**Fig. 2**). MR angiography (MRA) could also be use to evaluate for proximal vessel thrombus,[11] though accessibility, scan time, and patient-screening constraints may somewhat limit the feasibility of MRA.

A more experimental imaging component of acute stroke evaluation, perfusion imaging, may also be useful in the evaluation before intervention. While CT or MRI may show the already infarcted tissue, and CTA or MRA may show the site of an occluded artery, perfusion imaging can show the physiologic implications of the occluded artery. The pathophysiology of cerebral infarction is

complex, with a variety of factors in addition to site of arterial occlusion, such as cerebrovascular reserve and the abundance of collateral pathways. The concept of using perfusion imaging in the setting of acute stroke is to separate the completed infarct "core"—which is presumably irreversibly compromised—from the surrounding affected "penumbra"[12] or ischemic/oligemic tissue that can be salvaged (**Fig. 3**). The size of this mismatch is postulated to be an important factor in determining the risk or benefit of intervention[13] and may lead to a better selection of

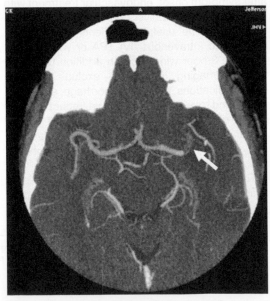

Fig. 2. CTA showing LMCA occlusion (arrow).

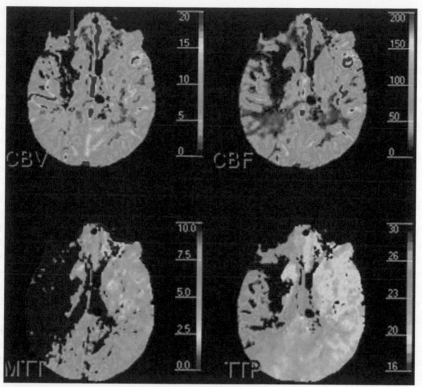

Fig. 3. Perfusion CT showing large portion of the right MCA (RMCA) territory, with prolonged mean transit time and decreased cerebral blood flow and a relatively small area of infarction, seen as decreased cerebral blood volume (*arrow*). This is compatible with a large area at risk for infarction in this patient with a RMCA clot.

patients, possibly expanding the window for intervention in the anterior circulation beyond the current 3 hours for IV thrombolysis, 6 hours for intra-arterial thrombolysis, or 8 hours for mechanical thrombectomy. The use of perfusion imaging has been included in the selection criteria for some trials (DIAS, DEDAS, DEFUSE, EPITHET, MR RESCUE), but there is little data on the role of perfusion imaging in clinical decision making.[14] While both CT and MR perfusion imaging are based on a similar theory and offer similar information, MR perfusion offers whole-brain coverage, while current CT methods offer only coverage of a portion of the brain contingent on detector number. On the other hand, CT is more accessible and has fewer contraindications. CT coverage also improves as the number of detectors on scanners increase.

A major issue with applying perfusion imaging is the complex nature of perfusion imaging. Unlike a CT angiogram or a diffusion sequence, a perfusion study generates multiple parameter maps, typically mean transit time, time to peak, cerebral blood volume (CBV), and cerebral blood flow (CBF) from dynamic CT or MR images following significant postprocessing based on bolus

tracking methods. These maps are produced by postprocessing the dynamic CT or MR images, using computer models based on indicator dilution methods similar to the thermodilution techniques used with a Swan-Ganz catheter. The accuracy of these maps is dependent on a number of factors related to the acquisition of the source images, such as patient motion and an adequate contrast bolus, as well as the how closely the data acquired for an individual patient adheres to the inherent assumptions of the computational models, such as the lack of contrast leakage from the intravascular compartment, appropriate arterial input function selection, and bolus delay and dispersion effects. Additionally, while each vendor uses similar methods, there are some variations between vendors.[15]

The mean transit-time map is the most sensitive[16] and is roughly inversely proportional to the local perfusion pressure. Time to peak is also sensitive, reflecting the delay of the contrast bolus caused by an upstream stenosis. Evaluation of CBV in isolation can be somewhat misleading, as in the initial phases of infarction the CBV increases, reflecting vascular dilation that occurs during cerebral autoregulation. However, CBV is the most specific, as areas with low CBV are likely to be already infarcted or will infarct. A CBF map would seem to be the most accurate single parameter, as the CBF is the "true" perfusion (ie, how many milliliters of blood per minute pass through a 100-mL volume of brain). While numerous articles have been written on the topic,[17–20] there is also no clear consensus on which map or combination of maps to use, or whether to use an absolute number or ratios. Thus, while promising, the use of perfusion imaging is yet to be proven to alter outcomes.[14]

CAROTID STENOSIS

Carotid artery disease is a common cause of cerebral infarction (**Fig. 4**A). While endovascular treatment of carotid stenosis remains controversial,[21] carotid artery stenting in patients who are at high risk for carotid endarterectomy is becoming more common.[22] In both, the measurement of carotid stenosis is a key factor in determining if intervention is beneficial. Although DSA was the method used for measuring of stenosis in the North American Symptomatic Carotid Surgery Trial (NASCET),[23] noninvasive imaging has moved to the forefront of carotid artery-stenosis evaluation.

Ultrasound is the most pervasive screening technique, however it is somewhat limited by operator dependence and variability in the velocity criteria used by different laboratories.[24] The main criteria for determining stenosis on ultrasound are based on velocities of the blood flowing in the carotid rather than direct measurements, as used on angiography. Other issues can limit carotid ultrasound, including incomplete imaging of high-carotid bifurcations and dense calcified plaque.[25]

MRA is also commonly used in the evaluation of carotid stenosis. There are a variety of methods of MRA, including two-dimensional (2D) time of flight, 3D time of flight, and contrast enhanced. While 2D time of flight is commonly used, it can be limited by motion artifact (**Fig. 4**B) and signal loss in areas of turbulent flow, and when vessels are oriented in the plane of imaging. For high-grade stenosis, time-of-flight and contrast-enhanced MRA (**Fig. 4**C) are highly accurate. However, for moderate stenosis the sensitivity of MRA is somewhat limited, with contrast-enhanced MRA being more sensitive.[26] An additional advantage of

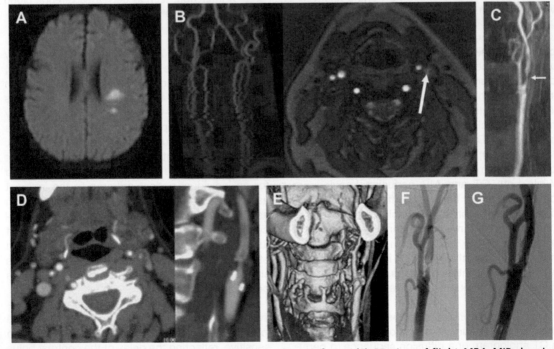

Fig. 4. (A) Diffusion-weighted MRI showing LMCA territory infarcts. (B) 2D time-of-flight MRA MIP showing typical motion artifact. Source images show high-grade left internal carotid artery (LICA) stenosis (*arrow*). (C) Contrast-enhanced MRA showing high-grade LICA stenosis (*arrow*). (D) CTA axial and oblique MIP recon showing high-grade LICA stenosis similar to the contrast enhanced MRA, as well as the location of calcified plaque. (E) CTA 3D volume-rendering image showing LICA stenosis. (F) DSA showing LICA stenosis similar to the CTA and MRA. (G) LICA after stent.

contrast-enhanced MRA is the ability to visualize the origins of the common carotid arteries and the aortic arch, areas that are not typically well evaluated on 2D time of flight.

CTA, similar to DSA, is based on contrast filling the vessel lumen but is noninvasive. Essentially a volumetric study that can be reconstructed in any plane, CTA can show the degree of luminal narrowing, morphology of narrowing, and composition of the plaque, including thrombus, ulceration, and calcification (**Fig. 4**D–F). NASCET-like measurements or simple diameters can be obtained from CTA data using measurement tools. Additionally, postprocessing techniques are available to measure stenosis, using a cross-sectional area that may better express the hemodynamic significance of irregularly shaped plaque[27] and may have superior interobserver agreement when compared with diameter measurements.[28] Measurement on CTA can be somewhat limited where there are dense calcified plaques if proper windowing is not performed.

In addition to measurement of stenosis, noninvasive imaging can also evaluate factors that increase the risk of carotid endarterectomy, such as stenosis in the high cervical internal carotid artery or in the common carotid below the clavicle, severe tandem lesions, or the presence of a contralateral carotid occlusion. Factors that are unfavorable for stenting (**Fig. 4**G) include irregular ulcerated plaque, tortuous arterial anatomy, dense calcification, and extensive atherosclerosis in the aortic arch.[29,30]

While measurement of stenosis is the prime factor used in determining the utility of surgery, plaque composition, a factor not included in NASCET, may also have prognostic implications. The presence of thin fibrous caps or intraplaque hemorrhage is associated with greater risk of rupture and can be detected on MRI.[31]

CAROTID DISSECTION

Methods similar to those used to detect atherosclerotic narrowing of the internal carotid arteries can also be used to detect carotid or vertebral artery dissection. Dissection can have a variety of appearances, from mild irregularity, intramural hematoma, stenosis, false lumen, or pseudoaneurysm.[32] Although the first-line treatment of dissection is medical, patients with high-grade stenosis, large pseudoaneurysms, or recurrent symptoms may be candidates for endovascular treatment to relieve stenosis and occlude pseudoaneurysms.

Both MRA and CTA can be used to evaluate for the luminal irregularities associated with dissection. MRI with T1 fat-suppressed images may offer a more sensitive evaluation of hematoma in the vessel wall. While the dissection-associated intramural hematoma is relatively isointense to adjacent tissue initially, within days the hematoma becomes hyperintense on T1 (**Fig. 5**), as the blood products convert to methemoglobin.[33] Vessel wall hematoma on CTA can be seen as a more subtle wall thickening. CTA has the advantage of higher spatial resolution, which can be especially useful when evaluating the vertebral arteries.[34] It also can give exquisite intraluminal morphologic

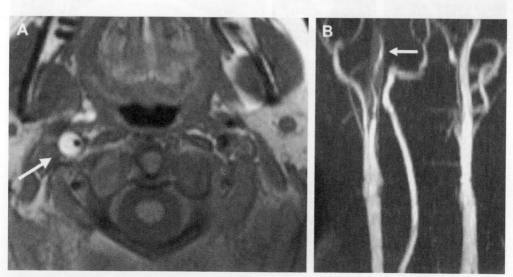

Fig. 5. (*A*) T1 fat-suppressed image showing T1 hyperintense hematoma in right internal carotid artery (RICA) wall. (*B*) MRA showing stenosis of RICA related to dissection.

information about the involved vessel, flap, and thrombus on the axial source data (**Fig. 6**).

POSTSTENT FOLLOW-UP

Once a carotid stent has been deployed, it is at risk for restenosis. MRA is at a disadvantage relative to CTA (**Fig. 7**) in this setting as the metal of the stent causes an artifactual loss of signal within the stent, related to the Faraday cage effect. CTA typically shows little artifact from stents and can well demonstrate the presence of luminal stenosis.[35]

ANEURYSMS

With the advent of spiral CT in the late 1980s, CTA emerged as an excellent noninvasive study to evaluate the morphology of the head and neck vessels (**Fig. 8**). With rapid improvement in both detector size and number, CTA has become a widespread study of choice in the initial detection and treatment planning of intracranial aneurysms. DSA with 3D rotational angiography (3DRA) is considered the gold standard[36,37] in the evaluation of aneurysms. However, CTA approaches the resolution of DSA/3DRA and offers other advantages. These include technical ease and speed of acquisition without need for

sedation, less pain, fewer resources required, and suitability for critically ill patients. CTA also is noninvasive, can image the bony landmarks and calcifications with respect to the enhanced vessels, and does not incur the 1.8% transient and permanent risk of angiography.[38]

DETECTION AND MORPHOLOGY OF ANEURYSMS

CTA detection of aneurysms has improved over time. A meta-analysis performed by White and colleagues[39] on initial studies performed with single-detector CTAs from 1988 to 1998 compared with DSA showed detection ranging from 61% for aneurysms 4 mm or less to 96% for aneurysms greater than 4 mm. Using 4- to 16-slice multidetector CT scanners, detection rates ranged from 74% to 91.7% for aneurysms less than 3 mm to 4 mm, and 92% to 100% for aneurysms greater than or equal to 3 mm to 4 mm.[40–45] Recent reports using 64-slice multidetector CT scanners suggest significant improvement in small aneurysm detection to well over 90%.[37,46,47] The improved detection of small aneurysms may be partially related to less-venous contamination afforded by the faster scanning technique available with the increased detector number.

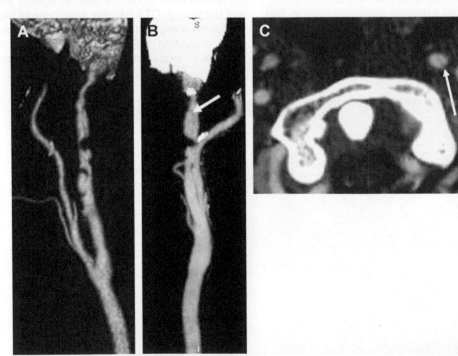

Fig. 6. (*A, B*) Volume-rendered and MIP image of an ICA with a dissection (*arrow*) secondary to fibromuscular dysplasia. (*C*) Axial source image from a CTA showing flap (*arrow*) in the ICA.

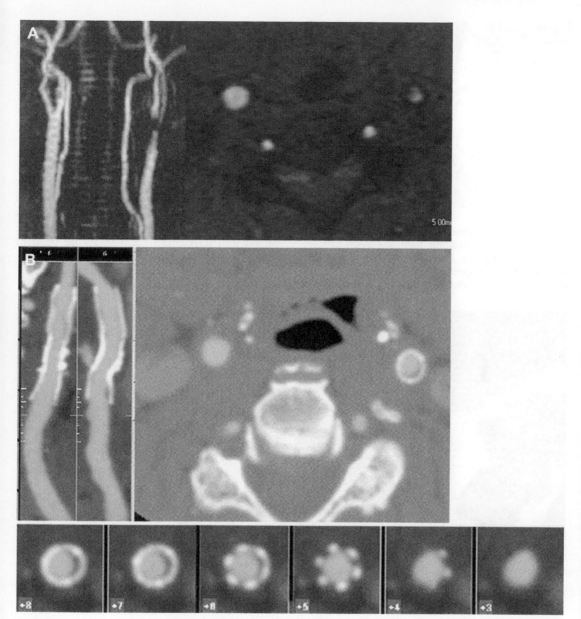

Fig. 7. (*A*) Two-dimensional time-of-flight MRA MIP and axial source image showing signal loss in the LICA at the site of the LICA stent, giving the appearance of stenosis. (*B*) CTA curved multiplanar reconstruction and axial images from the same patient as in (*A*), show only minimal stenosis present in the area of signal loss on MRA.

In addition to small size, multiplicity of aneurysms and those located in the periopthalmic and cavernous region (**Fig. 9**) had a higher incidence of missed aneurysms.[37,40,48] This appears to be secondary to proximity to bony structures at the skull base, as well as venous contamination. Small aneurysms at the level of the posterior communicating artery can also be confused with an infundibulum, and are also a source of possible false-negatives.[49] While the use of 64-slice multidetector CT scanners can decrease venous contamination, proximity to bony structures continues to be an issue. Various new bone-subtraction CT angiographic techniques are showing some promise in separating contrast-enhanced vessels from adjacent bone but need improvement for routine use.[50–52]

While the overall detection rate may be limited for very small aneurysms, in the setting of acute subarachnoid hemorrhage, sensitivity for the

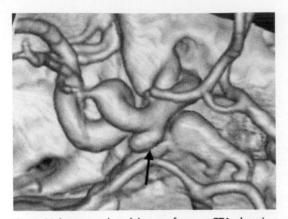

Fig. 8. Volume-rendered image from a CTA showing a posterior communicating level aneurysm (*arrow*) that was difficult to evaluate on a standard DSA because of the adjacent tortuous M1 segment of the MCA. Its relation to the clinoids is also well seen.

ruptured aneurysm is 99% to 100%, even when the ruptured aneurysm is less than or equal to 3 mm.[40,46,49,53,54] In addition to detection, morphology is also critical in the pretreatment planning of ruptured aneurysms. Morphology including lobe architecture, adjacent vessels, and neck-to-dome ratio are well evaluated, although CTA may slightly overestimate neck-to-dome ratio.[40,42,49] Papke and colleagues[55] demonstrated that morphologic depiction on CTA was able to correctly assess "coilability" in 93% (69 of 74) of target aneurysms with sensitivity, specificity, and positive and negative predictive values of 94%, 92%, 96%, and 88%, respectively. Hoh and colleagues[53] showed in a prospective clinical setting that CTA could successfully be used to triage patients. Treatment selection of endovascular coiling or surgical clipping was possible on the basis of CTA alone in 86% (93 of 109) of their

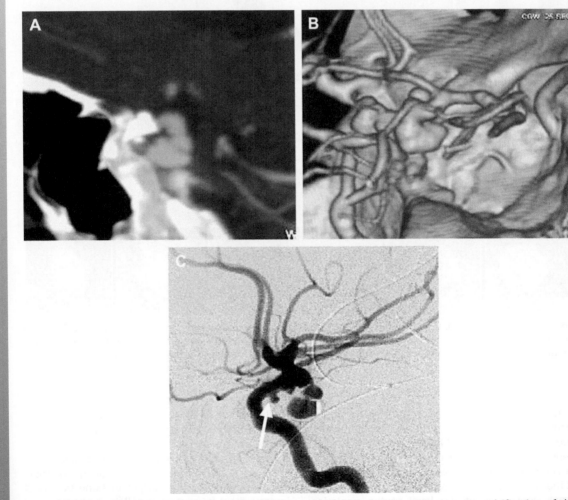

Fig. 9. (*A*) MIP image of supraclinoid irregular lobulated ICA aneurysm. Also note extensive calcification of the ICA, which may not be visible on DSA. (*B*) Volume-rendered image of the supraclinoid ICA aneurysm showing the position of the posterior communicating artery in relation to the aneurysm. (*C*) Lateral view from a DSA showing small cavernous aneurysm not visible on CTA (*arrow*).

patients with subarachnoid hemorrhage (SAH). Treatment selection based on CTA in other studies using a multidisciplinary team varies from 60% to 100%.[46,49,54,56] Three-dimensional workstations with real-time manipulation of large data sets allow numerous projections and postprocessing options from the submillimeter overlapping source images that allow standard and individual views to optimize aneurysm evaluation. While no one type of CTA data can give all aneurysm information, the two most common types of postprocessed images obtained in addition to the source data are MIP images and volume-rendered (VR) images, MIP images are more reliable for measurements of size, stenosis, and neck because they are less susceptible to distortion from artifact or windowing/leveling. VR images are best for overall 3D perspective of the aneurysm morphology and its relationship to adjacent vessels.

MRA using 3D time-of-flight techniques are often used for aneurysm screening purposes but are less useful in the acute diagnosis and pretreatment planning of aneurysms. Though detection rates are similar for medium-to-large aneurysms, detection of small aneurysms is inferior to CTA.[57–59] Decreased spacial resolution, signal intensity of blood products, and vascular flow influences inherent in the technique also limit evaluation of aneurysm morphology and associated vessels.

Finally, though CTA (less commonly MRA) is rapidly replacing DSA in the acute assessment of SAH, DSA is still needed when CTA (or MRA) is negative or when additional morphologic detail is needed. There also remains the question of what to do with the small number of unruptured aneurysms 3 mm or less that can be potentially missed. The relevance of these unruptured aneurysms varies as to whether they are present in the setting of multiple aneurysms where SAH occurred from a different aneurysm versus the isolated aneurysm in a patient who never had a SAH. The former group of aneurysms appears to be at a significantly greater risk for growth and rupture in the future, compared with those in patients who never had a SAH.[60,61]

COILED ANEURYSMS

Endovascular treatment of aneurysms with coil embolization is increasingly being used in place of clipping in the treatment of intracranial aneurysms, paralleling advances in techniques, catheters, wire composition, and supplementary equipment, such as intracranial stents. Recent data from the International Subarachnoid Aneurysm Trial has suggested that patients may have less morbidity and mortality when treated with coiling as opposed to clipping.[62,63] However, with coil embolization there is higher risk of rebleeding from incomplete embolization or aneurysm recurrence and continued surveillance is standard practice. While MRA is used less often than CTA for pretreatment planning of aneurysms, it is the predominant noninvasive imaging modality in the evaluation of coiled aneurysms. The high attenuation of platinum coils typically causes severe beam-hardening artifact locally on CT, obscuring the aneurysm site, adjacent vessels, and brain parenchyma, thus limiting the diagnostic value of CTA.[64,65] On MR/MRA, there is relatively little local magnetic-field distortion and subsequently little degradation of the adjacent signal. Compared with DSA, MRA sensitivity and specificity of source, and MIP data for detection of residual flow and recurrent aneurysm (**Fig. 10**) and patency of adjacent vessels is 80% to 100%.[66–68] In some studies, residual flow or recurrent flow was more frequently seen on MRA than on DSA,[69] though not with current 3DRA techniques. Earlier studies suggested a higher detection rate when contrast-enhanced MRA was used. However, more recent studies have shown conflicting results over whether there is significant added benefit of contrast-enhanced MRA over that of a high quality unenhanced 3D time-of-flight

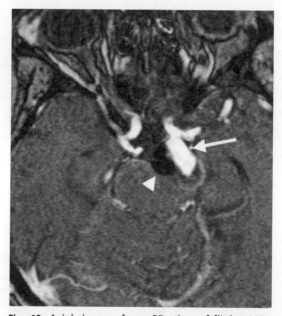

Fig. 10. Axial image from 3D time-of-flight MRA showing abnormal flow-related enhancement secondary to recurrence of left posterior communicating aneurysm (*arrow*) following previous coil embolization. The coil is seen as the hypointense signal medial to the recurrent aneurysm (*arrowhead*).

MRA.[70–72] It may be of benefit to do an immediate MRA follow-up compared with the DSA to see if MRA will be adequate for follow-up of coiled aneurysms, particularly in the presence of associated intracranial stents. Stents may potentially cause enough artifacts to cause either a false-positive stenosis within the stent, or obscure flow in an adjacent coil mass, erroneously suggesting complete aneurysmal occlusion.[65] As might be expected, artifacts are less for Nitinol stents with very little distortion of residual lumen as compared with those containing stainless steel. Contrast enhancement may show slightly better delineation of the vessel lumen.[73] Needless to say, in the presence of coils, CTA is very limited in the evaluation of associated stents. DSA/3DRA remains the most reliable method for follow-up of combined coiled aneurysm and associated intracranial stent patency in most cases.

POSTSUBARACHNOID HEMORRHAGE VASOSPASM

Once coil embolization or clipping has secured a ruptured aneurysm, patients with aneurysmal SAH remain susceptible to serious neurologic consequences from cerebral vasospasm, which typically peaks at 6 to 8 days after the initial hemorrhage. Symptomatic vasospasm is common, affecting 17% to 40% of patients following SAH, with approximately 50% of these patients developing infarctions.[74] To prevent infarctions, early detection of vasospasm is necessary so that maximal medical therapy or, in refectory cases, intra-arterial therapy with angioplasty, intra-arterial infusion of vasodilators or a combined approach can be performed.

Similar to imaging patients with infarction who may be candidates for intra-arterial intervention, detection of the site of arterial compromise is required. Transcranial Doppler (TCD) ultrasound is a commonly used bedside test used to screen for postsubarchnoid vasospasm. In the setting of MCA spasm, TCD has a high positive predictive value; however, TCD is not useful in other cerebral arteries.[75,76] While digital subtraction angiography is the gold-standard test used for spasm detection, noninvasive CTA can rapidly demonstrate the site and morphology of spasm with an

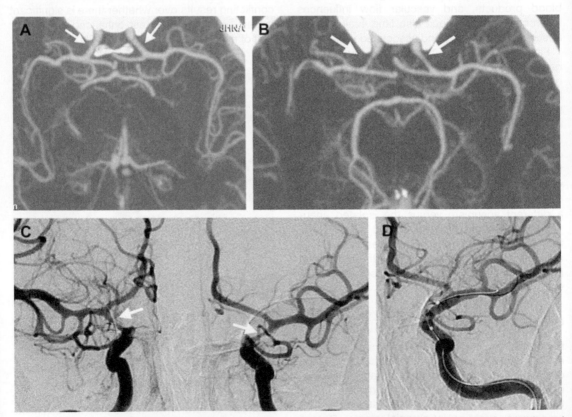

Fig. 11. (*A*) CTA at presentation, showing normal caliber distal ICAs (*arrows*). (*B*) CTA at day 5, showing bilateral supraclinoid ICA spasm (*arrows*). (*C*) RICA and LICA injections showing bilateral ICA spasm (*arrows*) similar to the CTA. (*D*) LICA after angioplasty.

accuracy of 87% and a negative predictive value of 95% (**Fig. 11**).[77] CTA, while useful, has some limitations, as sensitivity is higher in detecting spasm in the proximal vessels than in more distal branches, and CTA may be limited by streak artifact associated with aneurysm clips or coils.

The use of perfusion imaging, as with patients with embolic infarctions, may demonstrate areas where the cerebral perfusion is altered.[78] Perfusion imaging in conjunction with CTA may add additional information when the spasm is distal[79] or obscured by streak artifact, and may indicate the physiologic severity of the spasm. Perfusion imaging may also be useful in the follow-up of patients after treatment for spasm.[80] The impact of perfusion in post-SAH spasm management is not yet clear and may be more complex than that

for stroke. This remains an area of active research for the foreseeable future.

ARTERIOVENOUS MALFORMATIONS AND DURAL ARTERIOVENOUS FISTULAS

Proper evaluation of arteriovenous malformations (AVMs) and dural arteriovenous fistulas (DAVFs) require delineation of the origin, orientation, and course of feeding arteries and draining veins, as well as size, location, and morphology of the nidus. DSA/3DRA remains the standard for diagnosis of AVMs and DAVFs including carotid cavernous fistulas (CCFs). While the diagnosis can be made on MRI, MRA, and CTA, the lack of temporal resolution has significantly limited the data available on noninvasive studies. Small pial AVMs amenable to radiosurgery in certain cases may be adequately

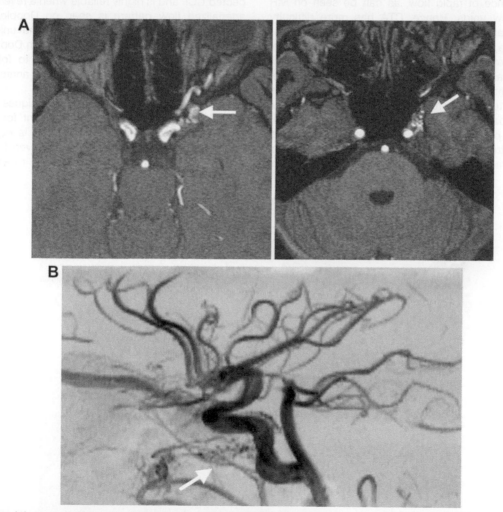

Fig. 12. (*A*) Two axial source images from a time-of-flight MRA showing multiple small abnormal arterialized vessels in the left cavernous sinus (*arrows*), as well as arterialized flow in the proximal superior ophthalmic vein in this patient with a dural type CCF. (*B*) MIP image from same study as (*A*) showing abnormal arterialized small vessels (*arrow*) in the cavernous sinus and enlarged arterialized superior ophthalmic vein.

evaluated and localized by MR and CT techniques.[81,82] However, these noninvasive techniques are generally not adequate at the present time for complex pretherapeutic embolization planning.

MRI and MRA can show abnormal flow voids in abnormal locations, suggesting abnormal shunting and arterialized flow, but complete identification of veins and the nidus is not optimal.[83] Abnormal signal in vessels is nonspecific and can represent slow flow or blood clot in various stages, even with contrast. Signal changes are further complicated after embolization. Though CTA has a slightly higher resolution than MRA, it relies on vascular enhancement from intravenous administration of contrast. CTA does not have the ability to suppress venous structures and does not have the ability to determine the presence of rapid flow, as can be seen on MR as flow voids. Hence, CTA has more difficulty separating arteries and veins.[84] In the parenchyma, this may occasionally cause confusion, separating a large unusual developmental venous anomaly from an AVM, or in the presence of a hematoma where normal vascular anatomy is distorted. One area where CTA may be helpful is separation of residual nidus from the embolized portion of the nidus, as glue material is better identified on CT than MR.[82,84] CTA is extremely limited in the presence of DAVFs

because the anatomy of the dural veins is so variable and the proximity to bone would be expected to yield a significant number of false-negatives. In this setting, MRI/MRA is likely to be more helpful for diagnosis. The exception may be in CCFs, where both MRI, MRA,[85] and CTA[86,87] have shown utility, though false-positives and -negatives remain.[88,89] Abnormal flow void on MRA (**Fig. 12**) in the cavernous sinus or early filling in the arterial phase of the cavernous sinus on CTA are highly suggestive. Secondary signs of an enlarged superior ophthalmic vein, proptosis, or enlarged ipsilateral cavernous sinus are supportive of the diagnosis. Direct high-flow CCFs, as expected, are easier to identify and characterize as compared with dural CCFs.[86] The use of Doppler ultrasonography can be used for screening purposes to confirm a suspected CCF and is highly reliable when a reversed arterialized flow pattern is seen on Doppler in addition to other secondary signs. The unique hemodynamic information available from Doppler Ultrasonography has also been used to follow CCFs after treatment,[90] though actual anatomic information is limited.

Newer 2D and 3D dynamic techniques for MRA[91–93] may offer some improvement for the future, especially where the diagnosis is equivocal,[91] but improvements in time resolved techniques are still needed. Preliminary research

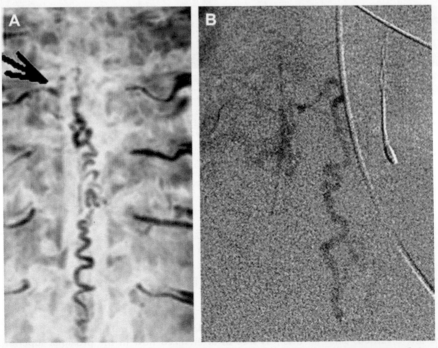

Fig. 13. (*A*) Contrast-enhanced MRA showing the radicular artery (*arrow*) that is the source of the DAVF in this patient. (*B*) DSA showing the same.

using dynamic CTA also suggests considerable promise both with the initial evaluation and in post-treatment cases, with sequential images at 0.5 seconds. However, this technique is currently limited because of radiation dose and limited scan range.[94,95]

SPINAL DURAL ARTERIOVENOUS FISTULA EVALUATION

Spinal dural arteriovenous malformations are a rare but treatable cause of progressive myelopathy. The suspicion of this diagnosis is typically raised on MRI of the thoracic spine, which usually shows swelling and T2-hyperintense signal in the thoracic cord. Additionally, dilated superficial veins may be seen on the surface of the cord. Spinal dural AVFs are thought to be acquired lesions, typically occurring later in life. The location of the fistula is usually adjacent to the neural foramen or within the nerve root sleeve, where a branch of the radicular artery forms a fistula with an intradural vein. This leads to venous hypertension and the associated engorgement of the cord.[96] While MRI may be suggestive or diagnostic of a spinal dural arteriovenous malformation, MRI is unlikely to show the level of the fistula. To treat the fistula either operatively or endovascularly, the site of the fistula must be known. Typically, this is accomplished with DSA, though both contrast enhanced MRA (**Fig. 13**) and CTA have found some success in localizing the site of the fistula noninvasively.[97–99] Locating the level of the arterial feeder or feeders may speed subsequent catheter angiography. Both MRA and CTA are somewhat limited by their inherent spatial and temporal resolution in detecting the smallest feeders, which may be seen on catheter angiography only.

REFERENCES

1. Rosamond W, Flegal K, Furie K, et al. Heart disease and stroke statistics–2008 update: a report from the American Heart Association Statistics Committee and Stroke Statistics Subcommittee. Circulation 2008;117:e63.
2. The National Institute of Neurological Disorders and Stroke rt-PA Stroke Study Group. Tissue plasminogen activator for acute ischemic stroke. N Engl J Med 1995;333:1581–8.
3. Smith WS, Sung G, Saver J, et al. Mechanical thrombectomy for acute ischemic stroke: final results of the Multi MERCI trial. Stroke 2008;39:1205–12.
4. Furlan A, Higashida R, Wechsler L, et al. Intra-arterial prourokinase for acute ischemic stroke. The PROACT II study: a randomized controlled trial.

Prolyse in acute cerebral thromboembolism. JAMA 1999;282:2003–11.
5. Adams HPJ, del Zoppo G, Alberts MJ, et al. Guidelines for the early management of adults with ischemic stroke: a guideline from the American Heart Association/American Stroke Association Stroke Council, Clinical Cardiology Council, Cardiovascular Radiology and Intervention Council, and the Atheros. Stroke 2007;38:1655–711.
6. Chalela JA, Kidwell CS, Nentwich LM, et al. Magnetic resonance imaging and computed tomography in emergency assessment of patients with suspected acute stroke: a prospective comparison. Lancet 2007;369:293–8.
7. Sims JR, Rordorf G, Smith EE, et al. Arterial occlusion revealed by CT angiography predicts NIH stroke score and acute outcomes after IV tPA treatment. AJNR Am J Neuroradiol 2005;26:246–51.
8. Powers WJ. Intra-arterial thrombolysis for basilar artery thrombosis: trial it. Stroke 2007;38:704–6.
9. Smith WS. Intra-arterial thrombolytic therapy for acute basilar occlusion: pro. Stroke 2007;38:701–3.
10. Lev MH, Farkas J, Rodriguez VR, et al. CT angiography in the rapid triage of patients with hyperacute stroke to intraarterial thrombolysis: accuracy in the detection of large vessel thrombus. J Comput Assist Tomogr 2001;25:520–8.
11. Schellinger PD, Fiebach JB, Hacke W. Imaging-based decision making in thrombolytic therapy for ischemic stroke: present status. Stroke 2003;34:575–83.
12. Astrup J, Siesjö BK, Symon L. Thresholds in cerebral ischemia—the ischemic penumbra. Stroke 1981;12:723–5.
13. Schlaug G, Benfield A, Baird AE, et al. The ischemic penumbra: operationally defined by diffusion and perfusion MRI. Neurology 1999;53:1528–37.
14. Provenzale JM, Shah K, Patel U, et al. Systematic review of CT and MR perfusion imaging for assessment of acute cerebrovascular disease. Am J Neuroradiol 2008;29:1476–82.
15. Boghosian G, Flanders A, Gorniak R, et al. Vendor variability in brain CT perfusion (CTP) calculations. RSNA 2007;SSC10–04.
16. Wintermark M, Fischbein NJ, Smith WS, et al. Accuracy of dynamic perfusion CT with deconvolution in detecting acute hemispheric stroke. Am J Neuroradiol 2005;26:104–12.
17. Schaefer PW, Ozsunar Y, He J, et al. Assessing tissue viability with MR diffusion and perfusion imaging. Am J Neuroradiol 2003;24:436–43.
18. Wittsack H, Ritzl A, Fink GR, et al. MR imaging in acute stroke: diffusion-weighted and perfusion imaging parameters for predicting infarct size. Radiology 2002;222:397–403.
19. Wintermark M, Reichart M, Cuisenaire O, et al. Comparison of admission perfusion computed tomography and qualitative diffusion- and

perfusion-weighted magnetic resonance imaging in acute stroke patients. Stroke 2002;33:2025–31.

20. Shih LC, Saver JL, Alger JR, et al. Perfusion-weighted magnetic resonance imaging thresholds identifying core, irreversibly infarcted tissue. Stroke 2003;34:1425–30.

21. Mas J, Chatellier G, Beyssen B, et al. Endarterectomy versus stenting in patients with symptomatic severe carotid stenosis. N Engl J Med 2006;355:1660–71.

22. Massop D, Dave R, Metzger C, et al. Stenting and angioplasty with protection in patients at high-risk for endarterectomy: SAPPHIRE Worldwide Registry First 2,001 Patients. Catheter Cardiovasc Interv 2008. Available at: http://dx.doi.org/10.1002/ccd.21844. Accessed December 1, 2008.

23. Barnett HJ, Taylor DW, Eliasziw M, et al. Benefit of carotid endarterectomy in patients with symptomatic moderate or severe stenosis. North American Symptomatic Carotid Endarterectomy Trial Collaborators. N Engl J Med 1998;339:1415–25.

24. Jahromi AS, Cinà CS, Liu Y, et al. Sensitivity and specificity of color duplex ultrasound measurement in the estimation of internal carotid artery stenosis: a systematic review and meta-analysis. J Vasc Surg 2005;41:962–72.

25. Back MR, Rogers GA, Wilson JS, et al. Magnetic resonance angiography minimizes need for arteriography after inadequate carotid duplex ultrasound scanning. J Vasc Surg 2003;38:422–30 [discussion: 431].

26. Debrey SM, Yu H, Lynch JK, et al. Diagnostic accuracy of magnetic resonance angiography for internal carotid artery disease: a systematic review and meta-analysis. Stroke 2008;39:2237–48.

27. Zhang Z, Berg M, Ikonen A, et al. Carotid stenosis degree in CT angiography: assessment based on luminal area versus luminal diameter measurements. Eur Radiol 2005;15:2359–65.

28. Bucek RA, Puchner S, Haumer M, et al. CTA quantification of internal carotid artery stenosis: application of luminal area vs. luminal diameter measurements and assessment of inter-observer variability. J Neuroimaging 2007;17:219–26.

29. Maldonado TS. What are current preprocedure imaging requirements for carotid artery stenting and carotid endarterectomy: have magnetic resonance angiography and computed tomographic angiography made a difference? Semin Vasc Surg 2007;20:205–15.

30. Roubin GS, Iyer S, Halkin A, et al. Realizing the potential of carotid artery stenting: proposed paradigms for patient selection and procedural technique. Circulation 2006;113:2021–30.

31. Honda M, Kitagawa N, Tsutsumi K, et al. High-resolution magnetic resonance imaging for detection of carotid plaques. Neurosurgery 2006;58:338–46.

32. Flis CM, Jäger HR, Sidhu PS. Carotid and vertebral artery dissections: clinical aspects, imaging features and endovascular treatment. Eur Radiol 2007;17:820–34.

33. Provenzale JM. MRI and MRA for evaluation of dissection of craniocerebral arteries: lessons from the medical literature. Emerg Radiol 2008. Available at: http://www.springerlink.com/content/k50u6677780477v7/fulltext.pdf. Accessed December 1, 2008.

34. Vertinsky AT, Schwartz NE, Fischbein NJ, et al. Comparison of multidetector CT angiography and MR imaging of cervical artery dissection. Am J Neuroradiol 2008;29:1753–60.

35. Jaff MR, Goldmakher GV, Lev MH, et al. Imaging of the carotid arteries: the role of duplex ultrasonography, magnetic resonance arteriography, and computerized tomographic arteriography. Vasc Med 2008;13:281–92.

36. Van Rooij WJ, Sprengers ME, de Gast AN, et al. 3D Rotational angiography: the new gold standard in the detection of additional intracranial aneurysms. Am J Neuroradiol 2008;29:976–9.

37. McKinney AM, Palmer CS, Truwit CL, et al. Detection of aneurysms by 64-section multidetector CT angiography in patients acutely suspected of having an intracranial aneurysm and comparison with digital subtraction and 3D rotational angiography. Am J Neuroradiol 2008;29(3):594–602.

38. Cloft HJ, Joseph GI, Dion JE. Risk of cerebral angiography in patients with subarachnoid hemorrhage, cerebral aneurysm, and arteriovenous malformations. A meta-analysis. Stroke 1999;30:317–20.

39. White PM, Wardlaw JM, Teasdale EM, et al. Can non-invasive imaging accurately depict intracranial aneurysms? A systemic review. Radiology 2000;217:361–70.

40. Yoon DY, Lim KJ, Choi CS, et al. Detection and characterization of intracranial aneurysms with 16-channel multidetector row CT angiography: a prospective comparison of volume-rendered images and digital subtraction angiography. Am J Neuroradiol 2007;28:60–7.

41. Dammert S, Krings T, Moller-Hartmann W, et al. Detection of intracranial aneurysms with multislice CT: comparison with conventional angiography. Neuroradiology 2004;46:427–34.

42. Wintermark M, Uske A, Chalaron M, et al. Multislice computerized tomography angiography in the evaluation of intracranial aneurysms: a comparison with intra-arterial digital subtraction angiography. J Neurosurg 2003;98(4):828–36.

43. Jayaraman MV, Mayo-Smith WW, Tung GA, et al. Detection of intracranial aneurysms: multidetector row CT angiography compared with DSA. Radiology 2004;230:510–8.

44. Teksam M, McKinney A, Casey S, et al. Multi-section CT angiography for detection of cerebral aneurysms. Am J Neuroradiol 2004;25:1485–92.

45. Tipper G, U-King-Im JM, Price SJ, et al. Detection and evaluation of intracranial aneurysms with 16-row multislice CT angiography. Clin Radiol 2005;60:565–72.

46. Agid R, Lee SK, Willinsky RA, et al. Acute subarachnoid hemorrhage using 64-slice multidetector CT angiography to "triage" patients' treatment. Neuroradiology 2006;48:787–94.

47. Pozzi-Mucelli F, Bruni S, Doddi M, et al. Detection of intracranial aneurysms with 64 channel multidetector row computed tomography: comparison with digital subtraction angiography. Eur J Radiol 2007; 64:15–26.

48. Anderson GB, Steinke DE, Petruk KC, et al. Computed tomographic angiography versus digital subtraction angiography for the diagnosis and early treatment of ruptured intracranial aneurysms. Neurosurgery 1999;45(6):1315–20.

49. Lubicz B, Levivier M, Francois O, et al. Sixty-four-row multisection CT angiography for detection and evaluation of ruptured intracranial aneurysms: interobserver and intertechnique reproducibility. Am J Neuroradiol 2007;28:1949–55.

50. Romijn M, Gratama van Andel HAF, van Walderveen MA, et al. Diagnostic accuracy of CT angiography with matched mask bone elimination for detection of intracranial aneurysms: comparison with digital subtraction angiography and 3D rotational angiography. Am J Neuroradiol 2008;29: 134–9.

51. Jayakrishman VK, White PM, Aitken D, et al. Subtraction helical CT angiography of intra- and extracranial vessels: technical considerations and preliminary experience. Am J Neuroradiol 2003;24: 451–5.

52. Tomandi BF, Hammen T, Klotz E. Bone-subtraction CT angiography for the evaluation of intracranial aneurysms. Am J Neuroradiol 2006;27:55–9.

53. Hoh BL, Cheung AC, Rabinod JD, et al. Results of a prospective protocol of computed tomographic angiography in place of catheter angiography as the only diagnostic and pretreatment planning study for cerebral aneurysms by a combined neurovascular team. Neurosurgery 2004;54(6):1329–42.

54. Westerlaan HE, Gravendeel J, Fiore D, et al. Multi-slice CT angiography in the selection of patients with ruptured intracranial aneurysms suitable for clipping or coiling. Neuroradiology 2007;49(12): 997–1007.

55. Papke K, Kuhl CK, Fruth M, et al. Intracranial aneurysms: Role of multidetector CT angiography in diagnosis and endovascular therapy planning. Radiology 2007;244(2):532–40.

56. Matsumoto M, Sato M, Nakano, et al. Three-dimensional computerized tomography angiography-guided surgery of acutely ruptured cerebral aneurysms. J Neurosurg 2001;94:718–27.

57. White PM, Teasdale EM, Wardlaw JM, et al. Intracranial aneurysms: CT angiography and MR angiography for detection-prospective blinded comparison in a large patient cohort. Radiology 2001;219:739–49.

58. Adams WM, Rogers DL, Jackson A. The role of MR angiography in the pretreatment assessment of intracranial aneurysms: A comparative study. Am J Neuroradiol 2000;21:1618–28.

59. Mallouhi A, Felber S, Chemelli A, et al. Detection and characterization of intracranial aneurysms with MR angiography: comparison of volume-rendering and maximum-intensity-projection algorithms. Am J Roentgenol 2003;180:55–64.

60. The International Study of Unruptured Intracranial Aneurysms Investigators. Unruptured intracranial aneurysms—risk of rupture and risks of surgical intervention. N Engl J Med 1998;339:1725–33.

61. Van der Schaaf IC, Velthuis BK, Wermer MJ, et al. New detected aneurysms on follow-up screening in patients with previously clipped intracranial aneurysms: comparison with DSA and CTA at the time of subarachnoid hemorrhage. Stroke 2005;36(8):1753–8.

62. Molyneaux A, Kerr R, Stratton I, et al. Internation Subarachnoid Aneurysm Trial (ISAT) of neurosurgical clipping versus endovascular coiling in 2143 patients with ruptured intracranial aneurysms: a randomized trial. Lancet 2002;360:1267–74.

63. Molyneaux AJ, Kerr RS, Yu LM, et al. International Subarachnoid Aneurysm Trial (ISAT) of neurosurgical clipping versus endovascular coiling in 2143 patients with ruptured intracranial aneurysms: a randomized comparison of effects on survival, dependency, seizures, rebleeding, subgroups and aneurysm occlusion. Lancet 2005;366:809–17.

64. Masaryk AM, Frayne R, Unal O, et al. Utility of CT angiography and MR angiography for the follow-up of experimental aneurysms treated with stents or Gugliemi detachable coils. Am J Neuroradiol 2000; 21:1523–31.

65. Wallace RC, Karis JP, Partovi S, et al. Noninvasive imaging of treated cerebral aneurysms, Part 1: MR angiographic follow-up of coiled aneurysms. Am J Neuroradiol 2007;28:1001–8.

66. Brunereau L, Cottier JP, Sonier CB, et al. Prospective evaluation of time-of-flight MR angiography in the follow-up of intracranial saccular aneurysms treated with Gugielmi detachable coils. J Comput Assist Tomogr 1999;23(2):216–23.

67. Westerlaan HE, van der Vliet AM, Hew JM, et al. Time-of-flight magnetic resonance angiography in the follow-up of intracranial aneurysms treated with

Guglieimi detachable coils. Neuroradiology 2005; 47(8):622–9.

68. Zoulin A, Pierot L. Follow-up of intracranial aneurysms treated with detachable coils: comparison of gadolinium-enhanced 3D time-of-flight MR angiography and digital subtraction angiography. Radiology 2001;219:108–13.

69. Yamada N, Hayashi K, Murao K, et al. Time-of-flight MR angiography targeted to coiled intracranial anurysms is more sensitive to residual flow than is digital subtraction angiography. AJNR Am J Neuradiol 2004;25(7):1154–7.

70. Farb RI, Nag S, Scott JN, et al. Surveillance of intracranial aneurysms treated with detachable coils: a comparison of MRA techniques. Neuroradiology 2005;47:507–15.

71. Pierot L, Delcourt C, Bouquigny F, et al. Follow-up of intracranial aneurysms selectively treated with coils: prospective evaluation of contrast-enhanced MR angiography. Am J Neuroradiol 2006;27: 744–9.

72. Anzalone N, Scomazzoni F, Cirillo M, et al. Follow-up of coiled cerebral aneurysms at 3T: comparison of 3D time-of-flight MR angiography and contrast-enhanced MR angiography. Am J Neuroradiol 2008;29:1530–6.

73. Lovblad KO, Yilmaz H, Chouiter A, et al. Intracranial aneurysm stenting: follow-up with MR angiography. J Magn Reson Imaging 2006;24:418–22.

74. de Oliveira JG, Beck J, Ulrich C, et al. Comparison between clipping and coiling on the incidence of cerebral vasospasm after aneurysmal subarachnoid hemorrhage: a systematic review and meta-analysis. Neurosurg Rev 2007;30:22–30 [discussion: 30–1].

75. Lysakowski C, Walder B, Costanza MC, et al. Transcranial Doppler versus angiography in patients with vasospasm due to a ruptured cerebral aneurysm: A systematic review. Stroke 2001;32:2292–8.

76. Fontanella M, Valfrè W, Benech F, et al. Vasospasm after SAH due to aneurysm rupture of the anterior circle of willis: value of TCD monitoring. Neurol Res 2008;30:256–61.

77. Chaudhary SR, Ko N, Dillon WP, et al. Prospective evaluation of multidetector-row CT angiography for the diagnosis of vasospasm following subarachnoid hemorrhage: a comparison with digital subtraction angiography. Cerebrovasc Dis 2008;25:144–50.

78. Binaghi S, Colleoni ML, Maeder P, et al. CT angiography and perfusion CT in cerebral vasospasm after subarachnoid hemorrhage. Am J Neuroradiol 2007; 28:750–8.

79. Aralasmak A, Akyuz M, Ozkaynak C, et al. CT angiography and perfusion imaging in patients with subarachnoid hemorrhage: correlation of vasospasm to perfusion abnormality. Neuroradiology 2008. Available at: http://www.springerlink.com/ content/d33287u45g715545/fulltext.pdf. Accessed December 1, 2008.

80. Hänggi D, Turowski B, Beseoglu K, et al. Intra-arterial nimodipine for severe cerebral vasospasm after aneurysmal subarachnoid hemorrhage: influence on clinical course and cerebral perfusion. Am J Neuroradiol 2008;29:1053–60.

81. Kondziolka D, Lunsford LD, Kanal E, et al. Stereotactic magnetic resonance angiography for targeting in arteriovenous malformation radiosurgery. Neurosurgery 1994;35:585–90.

82. Sanelli PC, Mifsud MJ, Stieg PE. Role of CT Angiography in guiding management decisions of newly diagnosed and residual arteriovenous malformations. AJR Am J Roentgenol 2004;183:1123–6.

83. Tanaka H, Numaguchi Y, Konno S, et al. Initial experience with helical CT and 3D reconstruction in therapeutic planning of cerebral AVMs: comparison with 3D time-of-flight MRA and digital subtraction angiography. J Comput Assist Tomogr 1997;21(5): 811–7.

84. Tartaglino LM, DeLara FA, Rosenwasser RH, et al. Evaluation of arteriovenous malformations with CT angiography. Radiology 1996;201(P):306.

85. Hirai T, Korogi Y, Hamatake S, et al. Three-dimensional FISP imaging in the evaluation of carotid cavernous fistula: comparison with contrast-enhanced CT and spin-echo MR. Am J Neuroradiol 1998;19:253–9.

86. Coskun O, Hamon M, Catroux G, et al. Carotid-cavernous fistulas: Diagnosis with spiral CT angiography. Am J Neuroradiol 2000;21:712–6.

87. Chen CC, Chang PC, Shy C, et al. CT angiography and MR angiography in the evaluation of carotid-cavernous sinus fistula prior to embolization: a comparison of techniques. Am J Neuroradiol 2005;26:2349–56.

88. Ouanounou S, Tomsick TA, Heitsman C, et al. Cavernous sinus and inferior petrosal sinus flow signal on three-dimensional time-of-flight MR angiography. Am J Neuroradiol 1999;20:1476–81.

89. Sakamoto M, Taoka T, Iwasaki S, et al. Paradoxical parasellar high signals resembling shunt diseases on routine 3D time-of-flight MR angiography of the brain: mechanism for the signals and differential diagnosis from shunt diseases. Magn Reson Imaging 2004;22:1289–93.

90. Duan Y, Liu X, Zhou X, et al. Diagnosis and follow-up study of carotid cavernous fistulas with color Doppler ultrasonography. J Ultrasound Med 2005; 24:739–45.

91. Akiba H, Tamakawa M, Hyodoh H, et al. Assessment of dural arteriovenous fistulas of the cavernous sinuses on 3D dynamic MR angiography. Am J Neuroradiol 2008;29:1652–7.

92. Gauvit JY, Leclerc X, Oppenheim C, et al. Three-dimensional dynamic MR digital subtraction

angiography using sensitivity encoding for the evaluation of intracranial arteriovenous malformations: a preliminary study. Am J Neuroradiol 2005;26: 1525–31.

93. Farb RI, McGregor C, Kim JK, et al. Intracranial arteriovenous malformations: real-time auto-triggered elliptic centric-ordered 3D gadolinium-enhanced MR angiography-initial assessment. Radiology 2001;220:224–51.

94. Matsumoto M, Kodama N, Endo Y, et al. Dynamic 3D-CT angiography. Am J Neuroradiol 2007;28: 299–304.

95. Yang CY, Chen YF, Lee CW, et al. Multiphase CT angiography versus single-phase CT angiography: comparison of image quality and radiation dose. Am J Neuroradiol 2008;29:1288–95.

96. Hurst RW. Vascular disorders of the spine and spinal cord. In: Atlas S, editor. Magnetic resonance imaging of the brain and spine. 3rd edition. Philadelphia: Lippincott Williams & Wilkins; 2002. p. 1829.

97. Saraf-Lavi E, Bowen BC, Quencer RM, et al. Detection of spinal dural arteriovenous fistulae with MR imaging and contrast-enhanced MR angiography: sensitivity, specificity, and prediction of vertebral level. Am J Neuroradiol 2002;23:858–67.

98. Mull M, Nijenhuis RJ, Backes WH, et al. Value and limitations of contrast-enhanced MR angiography in spinal arteriovenous malformations and dural arteriovenous fistulas. Am J Neuroradiol 2007;28: 1249–58.

99. Si-Jia G, Meng-Wei Z, Xi-Ping L, et al. The clinical application studies of CT spinal angiography with 64-detector row spiral CT in diagnosing spinal vascular malformations. Eur J Radiol 2008 May 20 [Epub ahead of print].

Techniques and Devices in Neuroendovascular Procedures

Kenneth M. Liebman, MD[a],*, Meryl A. Severson III, MD[b,c]

KEYWORDS

- Endovascular management • Embolization
- Stroke management • Intracranial stents
- Endovascular treatment of aneurysms
- Endovascular treatment of arteriovenous malformations
- Coil embolization

This article discusses the various techniques and devices used to treat cerebral aneurysms, cerebral arteriovenous malformations (AVMs), intracranial atherosclerotic disease, and acute cerebral ischemia by means of endoluminal approaches. Increased provider experience results in more successful and safer delivery of endovascular treatments. Success generates a greater interest in treating clinicians and in the industry, which helps to drive technologic advancements, which, in turn, broadens the use and improves the results of endovascular interventions. All these working in concert have advanced the field of endovascular neurosurgery to such an extent that there is almost no limit to where we can reach endovascularly and offer appropriate treatments. The field of endovascular neurosurgery is dynamic and continues to evolve rapidly, such that the techniques and devices used today are likely to be overshadowed and replaced by greater accomplishments in the ensuing years.

To comprehend the present and have a chance to shape the future, we study the past so we can learn from our forefathers' failures and successes. This allows us to understand why we deviate from some previous treatment strategies while expanding on others. The first description of an endovascular treatment was reported in 1904. Dr. James Dawborn,[1] a general surgeon, presented the results of his "starvation plan" for head and neck

malignancies at the 1904 American Medical Association. The procedure consisted of exposing the external carotid artery (ECA) and injecting Petroleum jelly and paraffin directly into the vessel. In 1930, Dr. Barney Brooks described the treatment of traumatic carotid-cavernous (C-C) fistulas by means of muscle embolization. The Brooks' procedure entailed exposing the common carotid artery (CCA), ECA, and internal carotid artery (ICA). Then, through a small arteriotomy, he would introduce a piece of sternocleidomastoid muscle and tie off the artery. The muscle would ideally flow into the high-flow low-resistance fistula.[2,3] In 1960, Luessenhop and Spence[4] first described the treatment of a brain lesion, a cerebral AVM. These surgeons exposed the CCA, ECA, and ICA, followed by directly introducing methacrylate and then plastic pellets into the vessel. The ICA was then ligated. The concept was identical to that described by Dawborn[1]; the pellets would preferentially flow into the high-flow low-resistance AVM.

The advent and improvement of the nondetachable and, subsequently, detachable balloons by Serbinenko[5] represented one of the first major advancements in the development of endovascular techniques. He developed and successfully used these latex balloons for the treatment of C-C fistulas. Debrun and colleagues[6] made minor modifications by introducing contrast into the

[a] Stroke and Cerebrovascular Center of New Jersey, Capital Health System, 1401 Whitehorse-Mercerville Road, Hamilton, NJ 08619, USA
[b] Department of Neurosurgery, Thomas Jefferson University Hospital, Philadelphia, PA, USA
[c] Department of Neurosurgery, National Naval Medical Center, 8901 Rockville Pike, Bethesda, MD 20814, USA
* Corresponding author.
E-mail address: kliebman@chsnj.org (K.M. Liebman).

Neurosurg Clin N Am 20 (2009) 315–340
doi:10.1016/j.nec.2009.01.002
1042-3680/09/$ – see front matter © 2009 Elsevier Inc. All rights reserved.

balloon and attaching an elastic band at the neck to prevent contrast leakage when detaching the balloon. This was one of the first times an endovascular treatment was offered to treat a disease process with lower morbidity and mortality than the surgical option. As a result, this new therapy was preferred over microsurgery in most centers as the treatment of choice for C-C fistulas. The modern beginnings and multidisciplinary expansion of the endovascular field corresponded to the development of catheters of variable size and stiffness. This allowed for more selective catheterization of vessels in various disease processes, enabling the clinician to deliver embolic agents with greater ease, safety, and effectiveness. As catheter technology improved, so did the need to improve the embolic material being delivered by the catheter.

There has been tremendous growth and advancement since the introduction of endovascular treatment in 1904. Dawborn[1] described a technique and used devices that were no more than an extension of everyday general surgery procedures. Today, we have specific devices for a wide variety of specific neuroendovascular procedures applied to cerebrovascular pathologic conditions.

FEMORAL ACCESS

When performing any endovascular procedure, the ideal artery to access, when feasible, is the femoral artery. It is technically easier and has lower complication rates than accessing the brachial and carotid arteries.[7] The artery is accessed by means of the Seldinger technique.[8] The original procedure has been modified to avoid penetrating the back wall of the artery. The right femoral artery is usually accessed, because most surgeons are right-handed and the angiogram suite is set up so that the right femoral artery is closer to the operator. Thus, he or she does not need to lean across the patient to perform the procedure. If the patient has a hemiparesis, the artery ipsilateral to the side of the weakness is accessed. A sheath is placed in the femoral artery, and the diagnostic and treatment aspects of the procedure are performed by placing a catheter through this sheath. The sheath eliminates the need for multiple transcutaneous catheter exchange, a process associated with morbidity.[7] The location of the femoral puncture site correlates with the potential vascular complications.[9] Too high a puncture (ie, above the inguinal ligament) increases the risk for retroperitoneal hemorrhage. Too low an entry increases the risk for pseudoaneurysm, arteriovenous fistula formation, hemorrhage, and arterial occlusive

problems. Using fluoroscopy, the femoral head is visualized and divided into four quadrants by imaginary lines.[7] The medial inferior quadrant is the site of entry into the common femoral artery (**Fig. 1**). Palpable landmarks include an imaginary line drawn from the anterior superior iliac spine to the symphysis pubis, which represents the inguinal ligament. The puncture site should be performed 1 to 1.5 finger breadths (1–2 cm) under this line, entering the skin at an angle of 45°.[8]

ANEURYSM TREATMENT

The earliest endoluminal treatments of cerebral aneurysms included directly introducing horsehair, silk-suture, electric current, and iron filings,[10–16] but Serbinenko and Debrun were the first to describe selectively delivering a latex balloon by means of a catheter into the aneurysm to accomplish endosaccular occlusion. This was the first attempt at true endovascular aneurysm management.[17] Unfortunately, the selective delivery of a detachable latex balloon in the aneurysm by means of a catheter was not overly successful. The inflation of the balloon resulted in aneurysm rupture, or, because the spherical shape of the inflated balloon did not correlate with the aneurysm shape, adequate occlusion was not obtained.[17] The development of the detachable platinum coil, introduced to the world in 1991 and approved by the US Food and Drug Administration (FDA) in 1995, revolutionized aneurysm treatment.[18,19] For the first time,

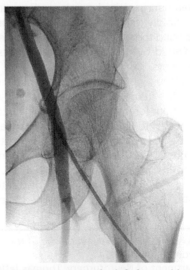

Fig. 1. Fluoroscopic image of a left femoral head with a 7-French sheath in position. Note that the sheath enters the femoral artery over the inferior medial quadrant of the femoral head approximately 2 cm below the inguinal ligament.

interventionalists had the ability to retrieve a deployed coil before permanent detachment. This allowed the endosaccular placement of coils with greater specificity and safety. In the initial studies by Guglielmi and colleagues,[18,19] the primary goal of the coil was to transmit a positive charge into the aneurysm, which would subsequently attract the negatively charged red blood cells, white blood cells, platelets, and fibrinogen, initiating thrombosis, termed *electrothrombosis*. Although the importance of electrothrombosis in initiating aneurysm thrombosis is controversial, the impact of the detachable retrievable coil on the endovascular treatment of aneurysms is irrefutable. There has been a proverbial explosion of coil types, catheters used to deliver the coils, and companies producing different coils since the inception of the first Guglielmi detachable coil.

The diagnostic and treatment procedures for ruptured or unruptured aneurysms are incorporated into one operation to avoid multiple anesthetic procedures, vessel catheterizations, and femoral artery punctures. The procedure is performed under general anesthesia with neurophysiologic monitoring (somatosensory evoked potentials [SSEPs], electroencephalogram [EEG], and brainstem auditory evoked potentials [BAEPs]). First, as previously described, the femoral artery is accessed, and a 7-French sheath is inserted and sutured in place. Baseline activated clotting time (ACT) is measured. The femoral sheath is attached to continuous heparinized saline flush (heparin, 4000 U, in a 1-L bag of saline). For elective cases, a heparin bolus is administered to increase the ACT approximately 2 to 2.5 times the baseline value. For ruptured aneurysms, heparin is delivered after the aneurysm dome and excrescence (if present) is protected.

Once the diagnostic angiogram is completed, a guide catheter is then positioned in the appropriate parent vessel. Through this catheter, microcatheters or other devices needed in the intracranial vasculature are passed. The guide catheter most frequently used at the authors' facility is a 6-French Envoy catheter (Cordis Endovascular, Miami Lakes, Florida). There are other guide catheters available that have a variety of different properties and shapes.

Under roadmap guidance, a hydrophilic glidewire is advanced and the guide catheter is then advanced over the wire to the appropriate position. Positioning the guide catheter as high as possible allows for greater support to the microcatheter. This is important when accessing more distal pathologic findings, especially when navigating through tortuous vasculature (**Fig. 2**).

The microcatheters used to access intracerebral aneurysms are wire-driven catheters. These catheters are not steerable but are navigated through

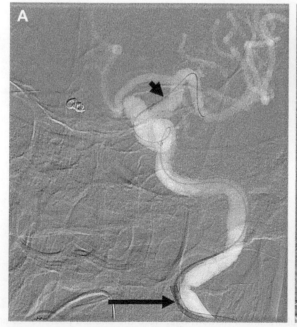
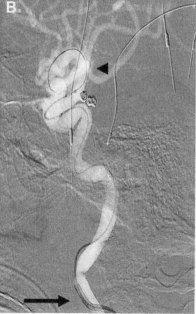

Fig. 2. The guide catheter is positioned just proximal to the entrance of the ICA into the petrous bone (*arrow*) (*A*). The guide is placed as distally as possible to provide support to the microwire and microcatheter (*arrowhead*) as they are advanced within the tortuous intracranial circulation to the site of pathologic findings (*B*).

the vascular tree by first manipulating a microwire through the arteries and then passing the microcatheter over the wire to the area of interest (**Fig. 3**). The microwires used have different properties. They are hydrophilic and have improved properties enabling a microcatheter to track over them through the cerebral circulation with greater ease. The microwire most frequently used by the senior author (KML) is the Synchro 0.014 wire (Boston Scientific Corporation, Fremont, California). This represents the OD of the wire minus 0.014 in. Some of the different properties of the microwires include different sizes, trackability, and torqueability.

There are numerous microcatheters one can use. Typically, the interventionalist becomes comfortable or experienced with a specific microcatheter, and this microcatheter usually becomes the "workhorse" for navigating through the cerebral vasculature and accessing cerebral aneurysms. The microcatheter most frequently used by the senior author (KML) is the SL 10 Microcatheter (Boston Scientific Corporation, Natick, Massachussets). The navigation properties of current catheters and microcatheters depend on the ability to fuse different polymers together so that the catheters possess different physical properties along their lengths. It is ideal for the microcatheter at the proximal end to be relatively stiff, creating a more "pushable" catheter or one with greater "torqueability" allowing easier navigation through the more proximal vessels. The catheter then progressively softens distally so it can reach the more distal vasculature with little vessel trauma or change in vessel geometry.[20] Some microcatheters and guide catheters have preshaped tips for greater ease of navigation and increased stability (**Fig. 4**). There is also currently available a "steerable" microcatheter offered by the Micrus Corporation, the Enzo catheter (Micrus Corporation, Inc., San Jose, California). As can be seen in **Fig. 5**, at the proximal end is a knob that, when turned, rotates the distal tip over 180° in one plane. This has the potential to help navigate through more tortuous vessels with improved stability and to gain access to pathologic findings at acute angles. Based on the authors' limited experience, the technology is still young in that this catheter is too large and cumbersome to access the distal vasculature. The microcatheters used have a different inner diameter (ID) and outer diameter (OD). It is important to understand that the size of the ID limits the size of the coils used or type of embolisate used. Once the microcatheter is in the aneurysm, the coil can be deployed.

The dimensions of the aneurysm, the size of the neck, and the ratio of the fundus to the neck are determined. The use of three-dimensional (3D) angiography allows for greater accuracy with these measurements. The 3D angiogram allows the interventionalist to inspect the aneurysm over 360°, assessing the shape of the aneurysm and, with greater accuracy, understanding the relation between the parent and branching vessels to the

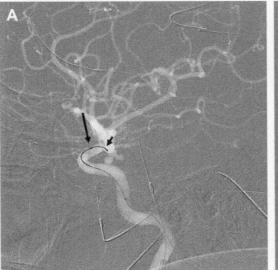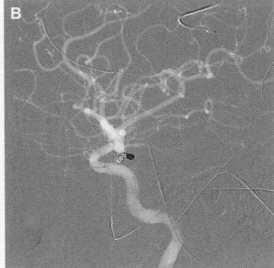

Fig. 3. This patient had a Hunt-Hess grade 3 subarachnoid hemorrhage. Note the bilobed posterior communicating artery aneurysm. (*A*) The microwire (*short arrow*) is advanced into the aneurysm, and the microcatheter (*long arrow*) is then "tracked" over the wire into the aneurysm. (*B*) The wire is removed, and coils are deployed through the microcatheter positioned in the aneurysm.

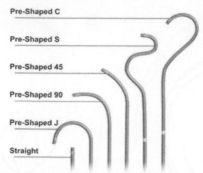

Pre-Shaped C

Pre-Shaped S

Pre-Shaped 45

Pre-Shaped 90

Pre-Shaped J

Straight

Fig. 4. Preshaped microcatheters and guide catheters offered by Boston Scientific Corporation for easier access and stability. (*Courtesy of* Boston Scientific Corporation, Inc., Boston, MA; with permission.)

neck of the aneurysm. This is the first step in determining whether the aneurysm is amenable to endoluminal treatment. Aneurysms that have a favorable fundus-to-neck ratio (2 or greater) or a small neck (<4 mm) can usually be coiled without the assistance of another device (ie, balloon remodeling or stent assistance).

The 3D angiogram also aids the interventionalist in obtaining a working projection to depict the relation of the aneurysm neck to inflow of the parent and branching vessels. This is the view that is used to catheterize and coil the aneurysm (working projection). Once the microcatheter is appropriately positioned in the aneurysm, preferably in the distal half, the coils are deployed. Depending on the shape and size of the aneurysm, the size of the neck, and the fundus-to-neck ratio, differently sized and shaped coils are used. Coils come in a variety of shapes (eg, helical, spherical), lengths (1–30 mm), diameters, softness, ability to "break" at different points, ability to maintain predetermined shape ("memory"), and bare platinum versus bioactive (**Figs. 6** and **7**). These traits give coils their different properties. It is important to remember the goal of the coil is to fill the aneurysm and block flow within it, thus promoting thrombosis and subsequent fibrosis within the sac leading to endoluminal healing.

A 14% to 34% incidence of aneurysm recurrence or coil compaction was reported in one of the largest single-center, long-term, follow-up studies involving bare platinum coils.[21,22] The goal of improving the long-term durability of this treatment led to the development of "bioactive" coils aimed at stimulating intra-aneurysm thrombus formation and denser scarring, reducing

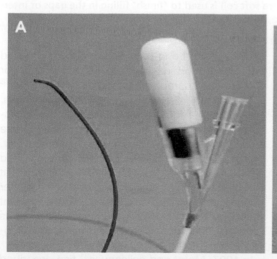
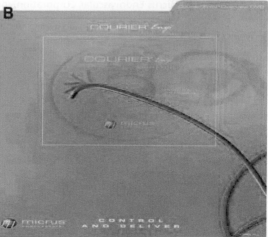

Fig. 5. (*A*) The Enzo catheter is an early-generation steerable catheter. (*B*) At the proximal end is a knob that, when turned, rotates the distal tip over 180° in one plane. This has the potential to help navigate through more tortuous vessels and gain access to pathologic findings coming off at more acute angles. (*Courtesy of* Micrus Endovascular Corporation, Inc., San Jose, CA; with permission.)

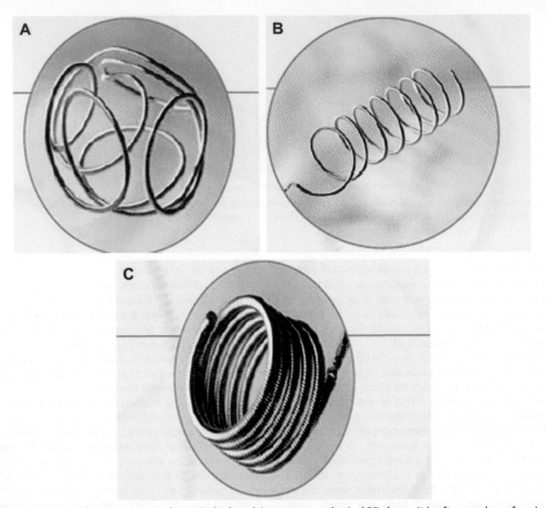

Fig. 6. (*A*) The coil has "memory"; when it is deployed, it assumes a spherical 3D shape. It is often used as a framing coil, especially with wide-neck aneurysms to help stabilize the aneurysm and coil mass. (*B*) Helical coil is often used to fill in the interstices or gaps between coils. (*C*) Extra soft coil is used to "finish" filling in the gaps or interstices. (*Courtesy of* Micrus Endovascular Corporation, Inc., San Jose, CA; with permission.)

the risk for recanalization.[23–26] The Matrix coil (Boston Scientific Corporation, Natick, MA) involves a platinum coil with an outer coating of a bioabsorbable polymeric material (polyglycolic acid/lactide), which, in swine models, showed acceleration of aneurysm fibrosis, neointimal formation, and increasing neck tissue thickness without parent artery stenosis.[25,26] Results of the human studies did not parallel the animal results and were somewhat disappointing.[24,27] The Cerecyte coil (Micrus Endovascular Corporation) uses the polyglycolic acid material on the inside of the platinum coils. The long-term efficacy remains to be seen. The third modified coil uses a different bioactive coil technology. The Hydrogel coil (Microvention, Aliso Viejo, California) consists of a platinum coil coated with a polymer that swells in contact with blood, increasing the coil volume

up to 11-fold. Long-term results show increased procedural morbidity and do not show superior outcome compared with the bare platinum coils.[28]

The treatment of aneurysms with wide necks, greater than 4 mm, or an unfavorable fundus-to-neck ratio (<2) has historically not had adequate results. The acute occlusion rates have been low, and subsequent follow-up has demonstrated high recurrence rates.[22,29–34] Attempts at complete aneurysm occlusion have led to higher thromboembolic complications in the parent vessel.[35] Thus, in the past, these aneurysms have not been considered appropriate for endovascular treatment.

In 1997, Moret and colleagues[31] first described the balloon remodeling technique performed in 52 aneurysms in 50 patients. These researchers obtained 77% total occlusion, 17% subtotal

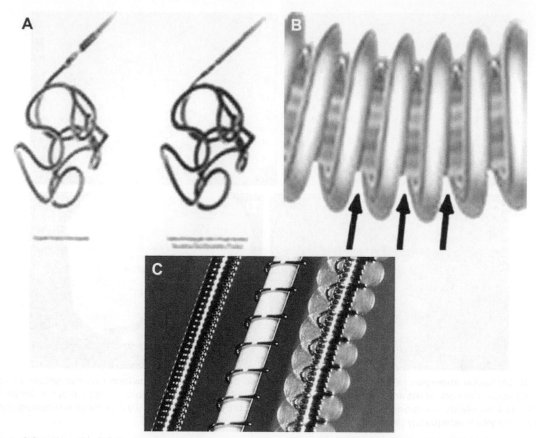

Fig. 7. (*A*) Coil on the left is a bare platinum coil, and the coil on the right is the Matrix coil. (*Courtesy of* Boston Scientific Corporation, Inc., Boston, MA; with permission.) This is a modified platinum coil with an outer coating of a bioabsorbable polymeric material (polyglycolic acid/lactide). (*B*) Cerecyte coil uses the polyglycolic acid material on the inside of the platinum coil. (*Courtesy of* Micrus Endovascular Corporation, Inc., San Jose, CA; with permission.) (*C*) The HydroCoil (MicroVention, Inc., Tustin, CA) consists of a platinum coil coated with a hydrogel polymer that expands when in contact with blood, increasing the overall coil volume. (*Courtesy of* MicroVention, Aliso Viejo, CA; with permission.)

occlusion, and 6% incomplete occlusion with 0.5% morbidity and no mortality. There have been other reports documenting excellent obliteration rates with wide-necked aneurysms using the balloon remodeling technique, but the procedure was associated with an increased risk for thromboembolic complications and periprocedural aneurysm rupture.[36,37]

As can be seen in **Fig. 8**, the microcatheter is navigated into the aneurysm. A wire-driven balloon catheter system is then positioned across the neck of the aneurysm. A coil is deployed into the aneurysm while the balloon is inflated. The balloon is then deflated. If the coil maintains its position and the interventionalist is pleased with the placement, the balloon is inflated and the coil is detached. This procedure is repeated until the aneurysm is protected. The balloon remodeling technique is a viable option for the treatment of these complex aneurysms, but there are inherent

morbidities associated with this technique. These include bilateral femoral puncture or a larger single femoral sheath, which increases risk for local femoral artery complications. As previously stated, repeated occlusion of the parent vessel increases thromboembolic complications and balloon inflation may cause intimal injury or rupture of the vessel or the aneurysm. There is also the potential for coil prolapse after the coil is detached and the balloon is deflated.

The FDA approval of a self-expanding nitinol stent in 2002 revolutionized the treatment of wide-neck aneurysms or those with an unfavorable dome-to-neck ratio. This stent is the Neuroform stent (Boston Scientific Corporation, Fremont, California).[38,39] The latest generation available is the Neuroform-3 stent. This stent has an open-cell design offering a greater ability to conform to the morphology of the arterial anatomy and aneurysm neck, theoretically reducing the risk

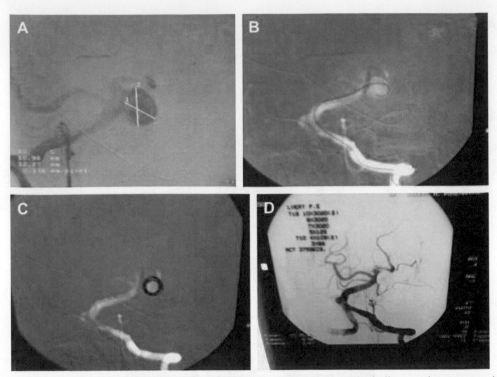

Fig. 8. (*A*) Basilar aneurysm. (*B*) Microcatheter is positioned in the aneurysm. The balloon catheter system is navigated across the neck of the aneurysm, and with the balloon inflated, the coil is deployed. (*C*) Balloon is deflated; if the coil maintains its position, the balloon is reinflated and the coil is detached. (*D*) Procedure is repeated until the aneurysm is adequately protected.

for coil prolapse behind the stent into the parent vessel.

In elective cases, the patient is pretreated with an antiplatelet, clopidogrel, for approximately 1 week before treatment. In emergent cases, the patient is loaded through an orogastric (OG) tube with Plavix (Bristol Myers Squibb, New York, NY, Sanafi—Synthelabo, Bridgewater, NJ) or a IIB, IIIA inhibitor. The Neuroform-3 device is a wire-driven delivery catheter with the stent and a stabilizer inside the catheter and with the stabilizer positioned behind the stent. The system is navigated across the neck of the aneurysm. Once it is in the ideal position, the catheter is slowly withdrawn over the stabilizer delivering the stent. Then, a wire-driven microcatheter is navigated through the cells of the stent into the aneurysm. The coils are then deployed. The stent acts as a scaffold, preventing the coils from prolapsing into the parent vessel (**Fig. 9**). A second stent was approved by the FDA in 2006 under the Humanitarian Device Exemption (HDE) Act. The Enterprise stent (Cordis Endovascular) is also a self-expanding flexible nitinol stent that, unlike the Neuroform-3, has a closed-cell design (**Fig. 10**). It is able to be retrieved before permanent deployment. The stent is delivered by a standard guidewire-driven

microcatheter. The microcatheter wire system is navigated through the vasculature across the neck of the aneurysm. The stent and the delivery wire are then loaded into the microcatheter. The stent is then deployed by withdrawing the microcatheter over the stent and wire. As stated, if the position is not ideal, the stent can be retrieved before permanent release. After deployment, the procedure continues as outlined previously. Because the stent is delivered by means of a wire-driven catheter, the intracranial vascular anatomy is no longer a limitation (see **Fig. 10**).[40] Onyx-500 (Ev3 Neurovascular, Irvine, CA) is another treatment option for wide-neck side-wall aneurysms and was approved by the FDA in April 2007. Onyx is a liquid form of ethylene vinyl alcohol (EVOH) dissolved in dimethyl-sulfoxide (DMSO). The DMSO dissipates when in contact with blood, causing the Onyx to solidify. Using Onyx for the treatment of aneurysms in human patients was first described in 2002. Mawad and colleagues[41] described the technique of first placing a balloon-expandable stent to reconstruct the lumen of the dysplastic vessel. The same balloon, which is DMSO compatible, is used to occlude the parent vessel when injecting Onyx in the aneurysm to prevent the Onyx from entering the artery. The

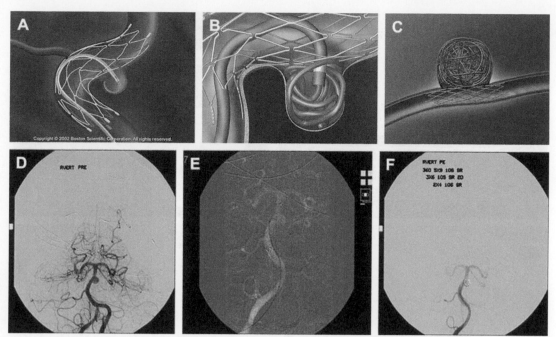

Fig. 9. (*A*) Neuroform stent has an open-cell design. It is deployed across the neck of the aneurysm first. Then, a microcatheter wire system is navigated through the cells of the stent into the aneurysm. The cells of the stent can accommodate a 2-French catheter. (*B*) Once the catheter is in the proper position, the coils are deployed. (*C*) The stent acts as a scaffold to prevent the coils from prolapsing into the parent artery. (*D*) Basilar trunk aneurysm with an unfavorable dome-to-neck ratio. (*E*) NF3 stent has been deployed. Under a new roadmap, an SL 10 microcatheter and Synchro 0.014 wire are navigated through the stent cell into the aneurysm. (*F*) Posttreatment controlled angiogram shows the aneurysm protected.

balloon also acts as a barrier to avoid the migration of the Onyx. It was a novel approach to treating a type of aneurysm that carries a significant challenge to the surgeon and interventionalist. The current technique is described without using an endovascular stent. As can be seen in **Fig. 11**, the microcatheter is positioned in the aneurysm. A second balloon-tipped microcatheter is positioned across the neck, and the DMSO-compatible balloon is inflated. Contrast is injected through the microcatheter to make sure there is an adequate seal across the neck to reduce the risk for Onyx entering the parent vessel. Long-term results using this agent for the treatment of aneurysms are yet to be determined.

ARTERIOVENOUS MALFORMATION TREATMENT

The morbidity of the procedure described by Luessenhop and Spence's[4] first attempts at AVM embolization is rather obvious, introducing the embolisates so far proximal in such a nonselective manner. Doppman and colleagues[42] were the first to describe the importance of embolizing as far distal in the arterial pedicle as safely possible. This decreases the possibility of the pedicle reconstituting more distal when occluded more proximal. Microcatheter development was imperative to access the distal vasculature safely and introduce the embolic material as selectively as possible. The early microcatheters had a small balloon mounted to the distal tip. With the balloon inflated, the blood flow would advance the catheter as far distal as the fourth- and fifth-order cerebral branches.[43] The catheter would selectively flow to the high flow low-resistance AVM. There was a limit in the ability to navigate through tortuous vessels, and these microcatheters were unreliable in their selective ability.

The current microcatheters used for endovascular treatment of AVMs are coated hydrophilic catheters that are flow directed and wire supported. This allows one to gain access almost anywhere in the vascular tree as long as the vessel and catheter lumen correlate. The embolic material can be delivered with improved selectivity, greater ease, and reduced morbidity. Because the procedure is performed with lower morbidity, the use or goal of endovascular treatment is broadened. The goal of neuroendovascular therapy with regard to AVM management depends on the overall treatment plan and is usually incorporated in a multimodal fashion. The most common use is as a precursor to surgical extirpation to reduce

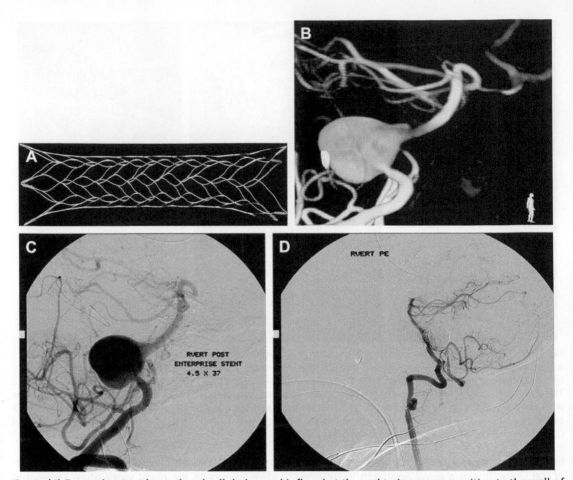

Fig. 10. (*A*) Enterprise stent has a closed-cell design and is flared at the end to improve apposition to the wall of the artery. (*B*) Giant vertebrobasilar (V-B) junction aneurysm with a dysplastic vertebral artery. (*C*) Angiogram is performed immediately after the stent is deployed to confirm proper positioning, no vessel injury, and no evidence of thrombotic complications. (*D*) Posttreatment controlled angiogram.

the potential for intraoperative blood loss and improve the ease of resection, thus reducing the potential for surgical morbidity. It can also be used as an adjunct to stereotactic radiosurgery. With the permanence of the embolisates used and the improved ability to access feeding pedicles, endovascular cure is more readily possible. Its use for palliative care is the most controversial, targeting the part of the AVM that has the greatest risk for bleeding or to reduce the shunt effect.

Before Surgery

The most common use for AVM embolization is as an adjunct to surgical extirpation. The aim of the procedure is to reduce blood supply to the lesion, reducing the technical difficulty of the operation. The interventionalist usually targets the deeper arterial pedicles, those that are more difficult to control surgically. Multiple studies, including the authors' own experience, illustrate the usefulness

of embolization in reducing the morbidity of surgical AVM resection.[44,45]

Before Radiosurgery

The goal of embolization before planned radiosurgery is not as well defined and is somewhat controversial. One of the strategies behind endovascular management is to reduce the size of the AVM to make it more amenable to radiosurgical treatment. The data to support the effectiveness of this approach are conflicting, but it is still commonly used. To simplify, the success of radiosurgery is directly proportional to the dose of radiation administered and inversely proportional to the volume of the lesion. Thus, the embolization procedure can theoretically reduce the volume of the AVM to a size that increases the effectiveness of radiosurgery. One challenge with this approach is that when embolizing the arterial pedicles and associated portions of the nidus, the embolized

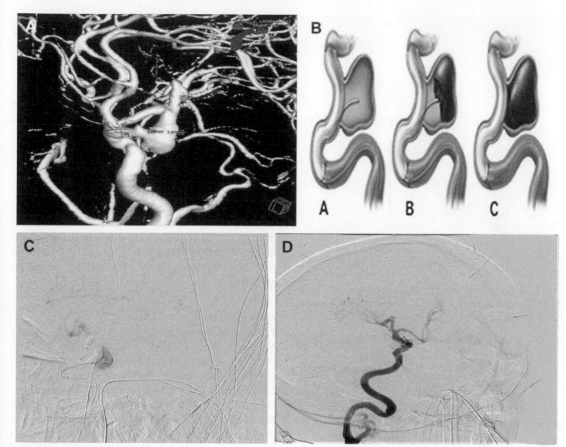

Fig. 11. (*A*) Dysplastic fusiform dorsal wall ICA aneurysm. (*B*) Cartoon representation of the procedure. The DMSO-compatible balloon is inflated across the neck of the aneurysm. (*C*) Contrast is injected through the microcatheter to confirm an adequate seal, as illustrated. The Onyx is then injected through the DMSO-compatible microcatheter. (*D*) Balloon can be deflated periodically and angiograms performed to assess the aneurysm occlusion. The procedure is repeated until the aneurysm is adequately protected.

portion of the AVM is within the volume of the AVM, and thus within the radiosurgical target. The embolization creates a "punched-out" area in the target but does not truly reduce the overall volume targeted (**Fig. 12**).

An additional goal of preradiosurgery embolization is to occlude the components that predispose the AVM to more acute hemorrhage, targeting pedicles with flow-related aneurysms or those that feed portions of the AVM with intranidal aneurysms. The interventionalist can also ablate the fistulous or high-flow shunting portions of the AVM, which tend to be more resistant to radiation treatment.[46] There is a latency of approximately 24 to 36 months for the radiosurgery treatment to take effect; thus, it does not offer immediate protection from possible AVM hemorrhage.

Curative

Much of the older literature quotes a 10% to 15% cure rate with endovascular management[47,48] and

parallels the authors' own earlier experience. As documented by Frizzel and Fisher,[47] a cure rate of 5% to 18% was reported in a review of 1246 patients in 32 series. The earlier studies, including the authors' own experience, suffered from referral bias, because, historically, embolization was used as an adjunct to other treatments; thus, those patients referred for endovascular treatment had complex AVMs that likely could not be managed with single-modality treatment. As can be seen in other studies, the cure rate has been shown to be much higher if AVMs with specific angiographic features are subclassified. These features include the following:

> AVMs fed by pedicles that can be accessed by a microcatheter and are not en passant vessels (a vessel that courses adjacent to the AVM and gives rise to small, serpiginous, side-branch vessels that feed into the AVM)

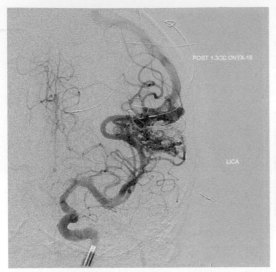

Fig. 12. Anteroposterior view of a left temporoparietal AVM. Onyx has been injected; however, there is still nidal filling around the site of embolization.

A single nidus that is more fistulous than plexiform

AVMs fed by three or less arterial pedicles or smaller than 3 cm in size

With these features, the cure rate has been recorded to be 31% to 73%.[48–50]

Palliative

This is the most controversial use of this treatment. The AVM being treated is likely not to be cured by surgery, radiosurgery, embolization, or a combination of these. The interventionalist approaches the endovascular procedure with the goal of occluding that portion of the AVM that is "symptomatic" and is the likely site or cause of recurrent hemorrhage or future hemorrhage. Partial embolization or occluding the fistulous portion (if present) can reduce the arteriovenous shunt, thereby decreasing the amount of "steal" or venous hypertension associated with the lesion. This has been reported to promote clinical improvement. Al-Yamany and colleagues[51] described the halting of the progression of neurologic symptoms in more than 90% of their patients who underwent partial embolization. There are various angiographic features that are likely to be the source of initial or recurrent hemorrhage or to predispose the AVM to bleed. One may target the pedicle that feeds the portion of the AVM with an intranidal aneurysm, and this may reduce the risk for bleeding. Meisel and colleagues[52] reported on partial embolization of "incurable" AVMs in 450 patients with high-risk features identified on angiography. They reported a reduction of the annual hemorrhage rate from 8.9% to 3.6% after partial embolization of the angiographically high-risk features.

Evidence to the contrary has been reported, documenting an increased risk for hemorrhage with partial endovascular treatment. Miyomoto and colleagues[53] reported on their series of patients who underwent partial embolization, documenting a 2.6% hemorrhage risk in the untreated group and a 14.6% risk in the partially treated patients. Kwon and colleagues[54] reported a 45.5% rate of hemorrhage in the partially embolized group as compared with a 25% rate in the conservatively managed group. Although using endovascular management as a palliative treatment is controversial, the authors do believe there is a role of targeting those angiographic features that are the likely source of current or future bleeding.

Embolisates

Particles Many different particles have been used for AVM embolization, with the more recently refined particles being polyvinyl alcohol (PVA; Contour Embolization Particles; Boston Scientific Corporation, Cork, Ireland) and microspheres (embospheres; EmboGold Microspheres; BioSphere Medical, Inc., Rockland, Massachusetts). The catheters required to inject these particles must have an ID large enough to deliver the PVA and embospheres without obstructing the lumen. These are larger and stiffer catheters than those needed for the delivery of liquid embolic agents. The catheters are wire driven with few flow-directed properties. These qualities make the ability to navigate the microcatheter through the distal friable vessels more difficult and hazardous. It is also relatively difficult to size the particles optimally to penetrate the nidus without occluding the arterial pedicle too proximally or passing through the nidus into the venous system. Embolizing with particles leads to higher recanalization rates as compared with liquid agents.[55,56] Because of this, the authors no longer use PVA or embospheres for AVM treatment.

Liquid Liquid embolic agents are the most widely used and most effective permanent agents for embolizing vascular malformations.[46] The two substances that are currently approved by the FDA are n-butyl cyanoacrylate (NBCA or Trufill; Cordis Neurovascular, Miami, Florida), a cyanoacrylate polymer, and ethylene-vinyl alcohol dissolved in the solvent base DMSO (Onyx; EV3 Neurovascular, Irvine, California). The original cyanoacrylate polymer was iso-butyl-2-cyanoacrylate. Its use was discontinued after studies demonstrated that it may have carcinogenic potential in animals. NBCA (Trufill) is introduced as a liquid monomer that polymerizes to an adherent solid when in contact with an anionic solution (ie, blood). The advantages of this substance are as follows:

1. Potential for penetration into the AVM nidus
2. Durability, permanently occluding the vessels treated
3. Delivered by means of a small, flexible, flow-directed microcatheter that can be safely and atraumatically navigated through the distal cerebral circulation

The disadvantages of this embolic agent are as follows:

1. It is difficult to control polymerization time.
2. The adherent nature prevents prolonged injection, with the possibility of gluing the delivery microcatheter in the vessel.

These disadvantages limit the ability to obtain significant nidal penetration with a higher chance of too proximal an occlusion or too distal migration with subsequent venous obstruction. A significant level of experience and expertise is needed to deliver this embolisate with optimal results.

The NBCA is radiolucent, but it is mixed with a radiopaque agent, usually ethiodized oil, such as lipiodol or Ethiodol (Savage Laboratories, Melville, NY). It can also be mixed with Tantalum powder (American Elements, Los Angeles, CA) to make it radiodense. The Trufill is prepackaged with vials of NBCA and Ethiodol. The mixing and diluting of NBCA not only make it radiopaque but alter its polymerization time. The more dilute the NBCA, the longer it takes to solidify, penetrating deeper into the nidus. The skill is in adjusting the concentration to get nidal penetration without too proximal or too distal an occlusion. Some researchers have found the Ethiodol-NBCA concentration to be inconsistent and have advocated diluting the NBCA with glacial acetic acid, finding that the polymerization rates are more reliable.[57] Acetic acid is radiolucent; thus, the mixture needs to be combined with Tantalum powder (also included in the prepackaged Trufill) to make it radiopaque. This powder makes the mixture more viscous.

At the authors' institution, the procedure is performed under general anesthesia. Neurophysiologic monitoring (EEG, SSEPs, and BAEPs) is performed during the procedure. Once the flow-directed compatible microcatheter is navigated to the optimal position, the NBCA and Ethiodol are mixed to the appropriate concentration. This is performed at a separate table to avoid contact with blood or any other ionic agent that can cause premature polymerization. The concentration is adjusted based on the flow dynamics and angioarchitecture depicted on the angiogram and microcatheter dye injections. Moderate hypotension (mean arterial pressure [MAP] of approximately 50 mm Hg) is then induced before glue injection. The catheter is then prepared by injecting 5% dextrose water through it. The glue is then injected under roadmap guidance. When appropriate, the micro- and guide catheters are rapidly pulled away from the site of injection to prevent them from being glued in place. The anesthesiologist may need to apply a Valsalva maneuver to the patient during the injection because this increases venous pressure, preventing or reducing the advancement of the polymerizing NBCA into the draining vein(s).

Onyx is EVOH dissolved in DMSO. The use of an EVOH copolymer for the embolization of AVMs was first described in the early 1990s.[58] This agent was approved by the FDA in 2005 for the endovascular management of cerebral AVMs. When Onyx comes in contact with an ionic substance, such as blood, the polymer precipitates by the diffusion of DMSO. The polymerization begins on the surface while the core is still liquid, creating a soft nonadherent plug. This quality creates a lava-like flow pattern within the blood vessels without fragmenting during injection. The advantages of this substance are as follows:

1. It is a nonadhesive and more easily controlled polymerizing liquid agent.
2. The nonadhesive property allows the operator to inject slowly with much greater control, with a significantly reduced risk for the catheter adhering to the injected polymer.
3. During the procedure, the operator can stop the injection periodically to perform controlled angiograms to assess the progress of the embolization.
4. Because of the lava-like flow pattern, Onyx has the potential to flow past previous areas of solidification into new parts of the AVM.
5. There is potential for improved intranidal penetration, minimizing the concern for too proximal or too distal an embolization.

The disadvantages are as follows:

1. The necessary microcatheter required for the injection of the Onyx is stiffer than the flow-directed catheters used with the injection of other agents. There is the potential for a higher rate of vessel injury while navigating this catheter.

2. DMSO has the potential for angionecrosis and vasospasm.
3. The EVOH-DMSO mixture is radiolucent and is mixed with the Tantalum powder to provide the radiopacity. Failure to mix or "agitate" the agent adequately may lead to sedimentation of the Tantalum powder from the mixture, which can result in suboptimal visualization of the Onyx during injection.

Onyx is prepackaged in ready-to-use vials. Each vial contains EVOH copolymer mixed with Tantalum powder and DMSO as the solvent for the EVOH. The polymer-to-solvent ratio comes in two different concentrations: 6% and 8%. The lower the concentration of the EVOH, the less viscous is the mixture and the more distal is the penetration that can be achieved. The viscosity of the Onyx comes as 18 or 34 cP (unit of viscosity) or Onyx-18 or Onyx-34, respectively. The Onyx-18, which is less viscous, is usually used for plexiform AVMs, whereas the Onyx-34, which is more viscous, is used for the higher flow arteriovenous shunts within an AVM or to embolize arteriovenous fistulas. At the authors' institution, the procedure is performed under general anesthesia with neurophysiologic monitoring (SSEPs, EEG, and BAEPs). Unlike the procedure for NBCA, hypotension is not induced and the patient is kept normotensive. The Marathon microcatheter (EV3 Neurovascular, Irvine, California), a DMSO-compatible microcatheter, is navigated as far distal and close to the nidus as possible with the use of a 0.010-in microwire. The catheter also has flow-directed properties, but it is important to remember that it is a stiffer catheter than that used with NBCA; thus, there is a greater potential for vessel injury. As with the other embolisates, superselective angiograms are performed to assess (1) where the catheter tip is in relation to the nidus, (2) the flow dynamics within the pedicle, (3) transit time from the arterial to venous phase, (4) that it is not an en passant vessel (a vessel that courses adjacent to the AVM and gives rise to small, serpiginous, side-branch vessels that feed into the AVM), and (5) the origin of branches feeding normal brain that could be compromised by reflux of the embolisate. The Onyx vials are on a shaker being mixed while the catheterization is being performed. The vials need to be mixed for at least 15 minutes, as described previously. The observed transit time helps to determine which concentration of Onyx is to be used (Onyx-18 or Onyx-34), as previously described.

Prior to embolization, microcatheter redundancy is removed by slowly pulling back on the microcatheter under fluoroscopic guidance. The catheter is then prepared by flushing it with saline to clear it of contrast. Then, DMSO (0.25 mL) is injected into the catheter to fill the 0.23-mL dead space of the catheter and to create a meniscus at the catheter hub. The Onyx is then injected with the first 0.25 mL injected over 90 seconds. The injection of the first 0.25 mL is slow because it is replacing the DMSO in the dead space, advancing the DMSO into the intravascular space. To eliminate the angionecrotic potential of DMSO, it needs to be delivered slowly.[59] The injection is performed under a new blank roadmap to ensure optimal visualization of the Onyx. As previously stated, because of its nonadherent nature, the injection is slow and controlled. The injection can be interrupted by intermittent angiograms to assess the progress of the glue cast and, if need be, can be continued. The initial infusion of the EVOH is continued until the mixture is seen refluxing around the catheter tip, and the infusion then is stopped for several minutes. A new blank roadmap is created, and the injection is resumed. Ideally, antegrade flow is re-established, and the Onyx progresses into the nidus. The infusion is again halted when reflux is visualized. This procedure is repeated until the desired effect is obtained or until no further reflux can be tolerated for fear of occluding a normal branching vessel. As compared with the process with NBCA, the microcatheter is removed by slow gentle traction. The traction is continuous, and, depending on the tortuosity of the pedicle, the length of time of the procedure, and the amount of Onyx reflux, different degrees of resistance are encountered.

Long-term data are being acquired, but until proved otherwise, like NBCA, EVOH should be and is considered a permanent embolic agent. Jahan and colleagues[60] reported no recanalizations in their series of patients imaged 20 months after embolization. To date, in the authors' experience, those patients experiencing a cure with Onyx embolization have not developed recanalization on 12-month follow-up angiograms.

ETOH is a sclerosing agent that results in permanent injury to the endothelial cell and, subsequently, permanent occlusion of the vessel. Because of the success in eradicating peripheral vascular malformations, interventionalists have advocated the use of ETOH for the treatment of central nervous system AVMs.[61] Because of the extensive risks, the high level of experience needed to use ETOH with safety, and the availability of other permanent embolic agents, there is general reluctance to use this agent for embolizing cerebral AVMs.

For larger AVMs, the embolization procedure is usually staged to avoid an abrupt shunting of blood into the adjacent normal brain that has impaired autoregulation. This can result in hemorrhage into the surrounding parenchyma, which is known as normal perfusion breakthrough. The number of pedicles accessed and the number of embolization procedures performed during each session depend on the preference of the interventionalist and the goal of the procedure. Although when staging the embolization process, the patient is obviously being subjected to multiple procedures and the associated morbidity, the staging process is encouraged. The authors stage the procedures approximately 3 to 4 weeks apart.

After surgery, the patients are monitored in the intensive or intermediate care unit with an indwelling arterial line for continuous blood pressure assessment. Mild hypotension (MAP <80 mm Hg) is maintained for 24 hours to minimize the risk for breakthrough hemorrhage. Dexamethasone is used around the time of surgery to combat the inflammatory response that may occur when using the NBCA. The authors do not routinely use anticoagulation during the procedure, except for the heparin, which is mixed with the saline bags that flush the catheter systems. The femoral sheath is removed the evening of the embolization procedure. The patient is usually discharged the following day.

ACUTE CEREBRAL ISCHEMIA

The epidemiology of stroke is sobering. An estimated 780,000 new or recurrent strokes occur each year in the United States, 87% (678,600) of which are ischemic.[62] Stroke ranks third in all causes of death behind heart disease and cancer.[62] The total cost of stroke in direct and indirect costs is $65.5 billion.[62] The number of stroke centers across the United States is increasing, as are the early identification, treatment, and referral to appropriate centers of patients who have this devastating disease. The number of patients reaching appropriate medical attention is growing, and coupled with the advancement of neuroendovascular technology, we are now uniquely positioned to provide real substantive treatment options for patients who have acute cerebral ischemia. As our technology continues to evolve, so should our ability to help this unique population.

To give the patient the greatest chance at neurologic improvement, speed of diagnosis and treatment is essential. Pre-endovascular treatments are just as important, if not more so, than the interventions themselves. Obtaining an accurate history and physical examination is critical. It is imperative to know if a patient has had previous vascular or endovascular procedures, which could alter the diagnostic and treatment plans. Additionally, the interventionalist must know what medications the patient has been taking or has been given, especially as they relate to the coagulation cascade. The physical examination is paramount to assess the patient's current neurologic status and National Institutes of Health Stroke Scale (NIHSS) grade. Clinical improvement since symptom onset may obviate the need for cerebral angiography, whereas deterioration may indicate the need for an immediate head CT scan to evaluate for possible hemorrhage, which would then contraindicate endovascular intervention. In those patients with a Glasgow Coma Scale score of 8 or less, prompt endotracheal intubation should be performed. Maintaining oxygen saturation greater than 90% in addition to mild hypertension is an important measure to help preserve the ischemic penumbra. Intravenous recombinant tissue plasminogen activator (rt-PA) should be given within 3 hours of symptom onset in those patients without contraindications, and strong consideration should be given to emergent cerebral angiography in those centers with intervention capability. In 80% of patients who have acute stroke, arterial occlusions are seen at angiography,[63,64] with the most common location being those of the middle cerebral artery (MCA).[64] The natural progression of MCA occlusion is notoriously poor[65]; however, the armamentarium with which we can combat intracranial artery occlusion is growing and with encouraging results.

Chemical Thrombolysis

The first major advancement in the treatment of acute cerebral ischemia was the FDA's approval of rt-PA to be given within the first 3 hours after symptom onset. The seminal study published in the *New England Journal of Medicine* by The National Institute of Neurologic Disorders and Stroke (NINDS) in 1995 showed that patients given rt-PA within 3 hours of symptom onset were 30% more likely to have a good outcome at 90 days.[66] These were encouraging results and led to the prolyse in acute cerebral thromboembolism trial (PROACT) I[67] and II[68] studies, which examined the safety and efficacy of intra-arterial prourokinase (proUK) delivery at the thrombus in patients who had acute stroke with MCA occlusion and had not been given intravenous rt-PA. PROACT I was a randomized, double-blind, controlled phase II trial of intra-arterial recombinant prourokinase (r-proUK) versus placebo in M1 and M2 occlusion. It showed a trend toward higher recanalization rates.[67] PROACT II was a randomized controlled, open-label, multicenter clinical trial with a blind follow-up. A total of 180 patients were randomized to receive intra-arterial r-proUK plus heparin (study group) versus heparin only (control group). The r-proUK group achieved recanalization 66% of the time versus 18% in the control group (P<.001) and had a modified Rankin score of 2 or less at 90 days in 40% versus 25% in the control group (P<.04), respectively, with equivalent mortality rates.[68] The researchers concluded that there was a 15% absolute increase in favorable outcome and that for every 7 patients treated with intra-arterial r-proUK, 1 would benefit.[68] This was the first study showing improved outcome with arterial recanalization. Although the treatment did not receive FDA approval, the results of the study were so compelling that a position statement by the American Association of Interventional and Therapeutic Neuroradiology (ASITN) was made suggesting that intra-arterial urokinase is an appropriate treatment and that, based on the location of arterial occlusion, magnitude of neurologic deficit and time to treatment were potential criteria to determine which patients should receive intra-arterial treatment versus the FDA-approved intravenous treatment.[69]

To deliver intra-arterial thrombolytics, the occlusive embolus must be localized. The presumed vessel of interest is imaged first based on the patient's presenting signs, symptoms, and physical examination findings. Once the affected vessel has been identified, a microcatheter of the operator's choice is positioned just distal to the embolus and rt-PA (2 mg) is slowly infused. The microcatheter is withdrawn into the embolus, an additional 2 mg is infused, the microcatheter is then positioned just proximal to the embolus, and rt-PA is slowly infused over 2 hours (or until the vessel has recanalized) for a maximum dose of 18 to 22 mg depending on the protocol followed.

The Emergency Management of Stroke Bridging Trial was a double-blind, randomized, placebo-controlled, multicenter phase I study of intravenous rt-PA followed by intra-arterial rt-PA versus intravenous placebo followed by intra-arterial rt-PA.[70] Treatments were performed within 3 hours, and 35 patients were enrolled. Although there were no differences in measured outcomes at 7, 10, and 90 days, the trial did show better recanalization rates in the intravenous/intra-arterial rt-PA group. The Interventional Management Stroke (IMS) study evaluated combined intravenous (0.6 mg/kg) plus intra-arterial rt-PA results against the treatment (rt-PA, 0.9 mg/kg) and control groups of the NINDS rt-PA study published in 1995.[71] There was no difference in mortality rates between the groups; however, the patients in the IMS study had statistically

significant better outcomes at 90 days compared with the patients in the placebo group of the NINDS study.[71] When compared with the NINDS rt-PA treatment group, however, there was no difference in 90-day outcome measures.[71] The recanalization rate in the IMS group was 56%, and those patients receiving intra-arterial rt-PA within 3 hours of symptom onset were more likely to have a modified rank in scale (MRS) score of 0 or 1 at 90 days.[71] The conclusion of the study was that intravenous (0.6 mg/kg) plus intra-arterial rt-PA was just as safe as full-dose intravenous rt-PA (0.9 mg/kg), and the investigators recommended a full randomized trial.[71] Currently, intravenous rt-PA is the only medication that is approved by the FDA for the specific purpose of thrombolysis.

Mechanical Thrombolysis

The prime goal of acute cerebral ischemic therapy is to restore blood flow as safely and quickly as possible. Chemical thrombolysis takes time to be delivered after the occluding thrombus is identified (as long as 2 hours); during that time, the ischemic penumbra and infarcted territories continue to expand. Resolution of the thrombus then depends on molecular interactions, with the greatest risk being that of hemorrhage from aggressive anticoagulation. Chemical thrombolytics are ineffective against many types of thrombi, including embolic calcific plaque and organized clot. The intuitively faster and potentially more effective therapy to effect vessel recanalization in almost any type of occlusion is that of mechanical thrombectomy. The devices currently in use that are approved by the FDA are the Merci Retriever (Concentric Medical, Inc., Mountain View, California) and the Penumbra System (Penumbra, Inc., Alameda, California). This technology is in its infancy, but great strides are already being made.

One of the first studies published regarding mechanical embolectomy was the Mechanical Embolus Removal in Cerebral Ischemia (MERCI) I study in 2004.[72] This was a phase I trial to evaluate the safety and efficacy of mechanical embolectomy. Thirty patients at seven US centers with an NIHSS grade of 10 or greater were treated within 8 hours of their symptom onset; none had received intravenous tissue plasminogen activator (t-PA).[72] Twenty-eight patients were treated with the Merci Retriever: 43% achieved recanalization with the device only, and 64% achieved recanalization with the device in combination with intra-arterial t-PA.[72] Fifty percent achieved a good outcome 30 days after the procedure.[72] The MERCI II trial was a nonrandomized, prospective, multicenter safety and efficacy study in patients ineligible for intravenous t-PA.[73] The Merci Retriever was deployed in 141 patients, resulting in 68 recanalizations (48%).[73] A MRS score of 2 or less at 90 days was obtained in 46% of the recanalized patients and 10% of the nonrecanalized patients (P<.001).[73] The mortality rate at 90 days was 32% in the recanalized patients versus 54% in the nonrecanalized patients (P = .01).[73] The MERCI II trial showed the benefit of timely recanalization on good neurologic outcome. The MERCI I and II trials compared the recanalization rates using the thrombectomy device with the 18% recanalization rates reported in the PROACT studies control groups. The success of the MERCI II trial resulted in FDA approval of the Merci Retriever for thrombolectomy in acute cerebral ischemia in patients ineligible for intravenous t-PA or in whom it had failed.[73]

In 2006, a study was published examining the effectiveness of intravenous rt-PA in conjunction with mechanical thrombectomy in recanalizing occluded intracranial vessels (Multi-MERCI trial).[74] This was an international multicenter, prospective, single-arm investigation of large-vessel stroke in patients who received intravenous rt-PA and did not recanalize or were ineligible for intravenous rt-PA. A total of 111 patients underwent thrombectomy: 60 (54%) were recanalized with the Merci Retriever alone, whereas 77 (69%) were recanalized using the Merci Retriever in conjunction with intra-arterial rt-PA.[74] This study showed the most promising results to date in efforts at recanalization. Outcome data at 90 days showed a mortality rate of 30.6% and a MRS score of 2 or less in 34% of patients.[74] Flint and colleagues[75] then examined intracranial ICA occlusion specifically in the MERCI and Multi-MERCI trials combined. Eighty patients with ICA occlusion were identified in the collected trials data, and the recanalization rates were 53% and 63%, respectively.[75] A MRS score of 2 or less at 90 days was obtained in 39% in the recanalized patients and in 3% of those not recanalized (P<.001), and 90-day mortality rates were 30% versus 73%, respectively (P<.001).[75] The final Multi-MERCI results comparing older generation retrievers with a newer generation, the L5, were published in February 2008. Recanalization rates with the newer device trended higher but were not statistically significant.[76] Morbidity and mortality data were not different from previously published reports regarding the Merci Retriever.

The Merci Retrieval System is produced by Concentric Medical, Inc. (Mountain View, California).[77] It is composed of three components: a Merci Balloon Guide Catheter, a Merci microcatheter, and the Merci Retrievers (**Fig. 13**). Once

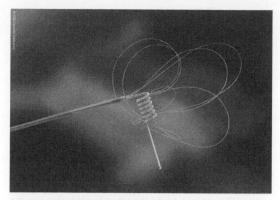

Fig. 13. L6 Merci Retriever. The helix and attached suture are designed to engage and extract intraluminal thrombi (*Courtesy of* Concentric Medical, Mountain View, CA; with permission.)

a mechanical occlusion is identified, and if it is located in the anterior circulation, the Merci Balloon Guide Catheter is placed into position in the ICA. The microcatheter is used in conjunction with a microwire; the wire is advanced distal to the thrombus, and the microcatheter is passed over the wire until it is also distal to the thrombus; and the microwire is then removed. Digital subtraction angiography (DSA) is performed through the microcatheter to evaluate the patency of the distal cerebral vessels and to confirm that the microcatheter is located immediately distal to the clot. The retriever is passed through the microcatheter until it deploys into the vessel, just distal to the thrombus. The microcatheter is withdrawn slightly until it lies proximal to the occlusion; gentle traction is applied to the retriever, allowing it to engage the embolus. The microcatheter is positioned just proximal to where the helix begins. The balloon is inflated to interrupt blood flow, and gentle suction is applied through the guide catheter with a large syringe to prevent the embolus from advancing further into the cerebral circulation. Continued gentle traction is applied to the retriever with careful attention paid to the retriever loops. As the proximal loops straighten, traction is maintained, and the tension of the helix, as it slowly resumes its shape, gently withdraws the embolus. The process is repeated until the retriever no longer straightens and can be removed through the guide catheter and evaluated for debris. The balloon is deflated, and DSA is performed to evaluate flow. If embolus remains, the procedure can be repeated multiple times until the desired vessel becomes patent. In the MERCI I and II trials, a total of six passes were performed. If the vessel was opened on any of the six attempts, the procedure was considered a success.[72,73] In the authors' experience, if the device does not recanalize the vessel, a different retriever may be chosen, such as one of a different size. If progress is not seen after the third pass, the authors frequently change mechanical thrombolytic devices. There are several types of retrievers with varying helical sizes, angles, and stiffness.

The Penumbra System is another endovascular device designed specifically for mechanical embolectomy.[78] The Penumbra System is designed to remove an occlusive thrombus by combining aspiration with mechanical disruption of the clot. The purpose of the initial trial was to assess the safety and efficacy of using this devise to open an occluded proximal vessel. This system demonstrated 100% revascularization in 23 enrolled patients in its phase I trial published in 2008.[79] Although it was not an outcome trial, the data at 30 days found 45% of patients had improved an NIHSS grade by 4 or more points or had a MRS score of 2 or less.[79] Because of the high rate of successful recanalization, the trial was stopped early and the FDA granted an HDE approval for the Penumbra System.

The system consists of a reperfusion catheter connected to an aspirator (continuous suction device) in conjunction with a separator to disrupt and remove the embolus mechanically. By means of a switch, the suction can be turned "on" and "off." While the suction is in the off position, the reperfusion catheter is positioned next to the proximal side of the embolus. The aspirator is turned on, and the embolus is partially aspirated into the reperfusion catheter. As this happens, the reperfusion catheter is momentarily obstructed. The separator, by way of a short distal wire with a proximal widening, dislodges and morselizes the embolic material, making it small enough to be aspirated into and through the reperfusion catheter. This process is repeated until the embolus has been completely removed and the vessel is recanalized. The device is currently offered in three different diameters (**Fig. 14**).

Authors' Management Strategy

A patient who has acute cerebral ischemia and is transferred to the authors' institution is brought directly to the endovascular neurosurgery holding area and examined by the treating physician. The entire treating team, consisting of the endovascular neurosurgeon; radiation technologists; and anesthesia, nursing, and neurophysiology providers, is present and prepared for immediate treatment. The time of symptom onset is confirmed, and an NIHSS assessment of grade is performed and compared with the score obtained by the referring institution. In patients who are markedly improving, no intervention is pursued. In patients who have not improved or have deteriorated, an emergent head CT is obtained. Findings of intracerebral hemorrhage or greater than one-third MCA territory infarction contraindicate neuroendovascular intervention. If these findings are absent, the patient is immediately placed on the cerebral angiography table. General anesthesia is induced, neurophysiological monitors (EEG, BAER–Brainstem auditory evoked responses (ABRs), and SSEPs) are placed, and the femoral artery on the symptomatic side is cannulated with a 7- or 8-French femoral sheath. Baseline ACT values are obtained at the time of sheath insertion, and heparin is given to achieve an ACT value of 200 to 250. The authors may choose an 8-French sheath so as to be prepared should they find carotid bifurcation or proximal ICA disease requiring angioplasty and stenting. MAP is maintained at 90 to 100 mm Hg throughout the case. The vessel of interest, based on the symptoms and findings, is studied first. When a thrombus is identified in a proximal vessel, mechanical thrombectomy is attempted (**Fig. 15**). If a more distal vessel is occluded, pro-UK is infused into the thrombus in an attempt to lyse the clot chemically.

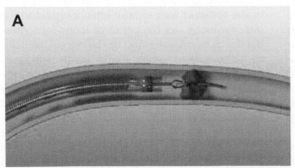 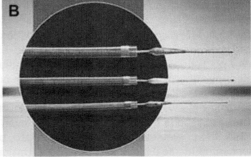

Fig. 14. (A) Cartoon representation of the Penumbra System engaging an intraluminal thrombus. (B) Penumbra System is available in three different diameters. Note the proximal widening of the separator used to morselize the intraluminal thrombus for aspiration (*Courtesy of* Penumbra, Inc., Alameda, CA; with permission.)

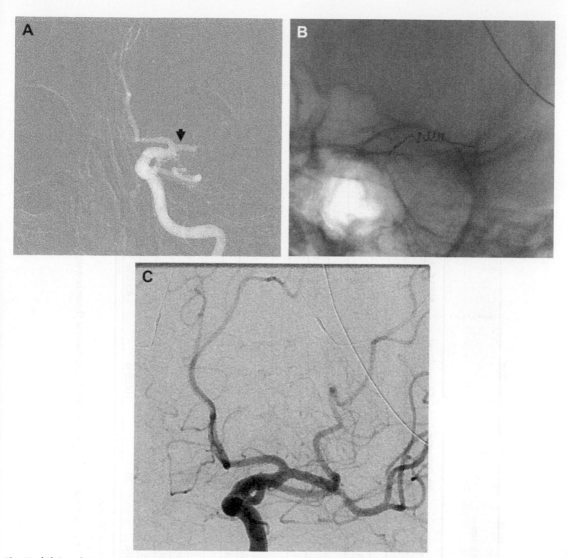

Fig. 15. (*A*) Roadmap angiogram shows M1 segment filling defect (*arrowhead*). (*B*) Merci Retriever extracts intraluminal thrombus. (*C*) Postembolectomy angiogram shows recanalization of M1 segment.

The authors often continue heparin for 24 hours, with a goal partial thromboplastin time of 50 to 70 seconds.

A brief summary of some of the various thrombolytic trials described in this article can be found in **Table 1**. In general, recanalization rates are better with the use of intra-arterial therapies whether they be chemical, mechanical, or both. In conjunction, neurologic outcomes seem to mirror the rates of recanalization, whereas mortality rates remain relatively unchanged. No individual therapeutic approach has proved itself to be superior to the others. Optimal outcome from acute cerebral ischemia continues to depend on early identification of stroke victims, timely use of intravenous rt-PA in indicated patients, rapid

transport to tertiary stroke centers, early cerebral angiography in nonimproving patients, and intra-arterial treatment by means of thrombectomy and thrombolytics. Aggressive postintervention medical and surgical management of cerebral edema is also critical in this patient population.

INTRACRANIAL ARTERIAL STENOSIS

Intracranial arterial stenosis is responsible for approximately 10% of all transient ischemic attack or acute stroke events per year.[80] Risk for recurrent stroke can range from 15% to 60% depending on the severity of the lesion.[80–86] As the population continues to age and life expectancy increases, the number of patients evaluated for symptomatic

Table 1
Summary of seminal studies in the treatment of ischemic stroke

Control Groups

		Control Method	No. Patients	Recanalized	MRS 0–1	MRS 0–2 Mortality Rate	Pre-NIHSS Grade
1995	IV t-PA (part II)	Placebo	165	—	26.0%	21.0%	14
1998	PROACT I	Placebo	14	14.3%	21.0%	43.0%	—
1999	PROACT II	Heparin	59	18.0%	25.0%	27.0%	—
1999	EMS bridging	IV placebo + IA t-PA	18	50.0%	33.0%	5.5%	—

Intervention Groups

		Intervention	No. Patients	Recanalized	MRS 0–1	MRS 0–2 Mortality Rate	Pre-NIHSS Grade
1995	IV t-PA (part II)	IV t-PA in 3 hours	168	—	39.0%	17.0%	15
1998	PROACT I	IA r-proUK	26	57.7%	31.0%	27.0%	—
1999	PROACT II	IA r-proUK	121	66.0%	40.0%	25.0%	—
1999	EMS bridging	IV t-PA + IA t-PA	17	81.0%	33.0%	29.0%	—
2004	IMS	IV t-PA + IA t-PA	62	56.0%	43.0%	16.0%	18
2004	MERCI I	Mech ± IA t-PA	28	64.0%	21.4%	36.0%	22
2005	MERCI II	Mech ± IA t-PA	141	48.0%	46.0%	32.0%	20
2006	Multi-MERCI	Mech ± IA/IV t-PA	111	69.0%	34.0%	31.0%	19
2007	Combined MERCI	Mech ± IA/IV t-PA	80	63.0%	39.0%	30.0%	20
2008	Final Multi-MERCI	New-generation L5	131	69.5%	36.0%	34.0%	19
2008	Penumbra	Mech ± IA/IV t-PA	20	100.0%	45.0%	45.0%	21

% MRS scores were measured at study follow-up, in most cases, at 90 days.
Pre-NIHSS refers to the median NIHSS grade before treatment.
Abbreviations: EMS, Emergency Management of Stroke; IA, intra-arterial; IV, intravenous; Mech, mechanical thrombolysis; r-proUK, r-prourokinase; t-PA, tissue plasminogen activator.

intracranial atherosclerosis should continue to increase. Maximal medical management of this patient population is notoriously associated with a significant stroke rate[84]; however, with recent technologic advancements in neuroendovascular technology, endovascular management is now a potential management option in those patients failing medical therapy.

The Stenting of Symptomatic Atherosclerotic Lesions in Vertebral or Intracranial Arteries (SSYLVIA) trial published in 2004 was the first to examine arterial stenting as a management option in patients who have symptomatic intracranial stenosis.[87] The Neurolink stent (Guidant Corporation, Indianapolis, IN) was successfully deployed in 58 patients; all had a single target lesion with 50% or greater stenosis. The recurrence of 50% or greater stenosis was 35% at 6 months, and the stroke rate at greater than 30 days was 7.3%.[87] This stent is no longer available.

The Wingspan stent (Boston Scientific Corporation, Fremont, California) is a self-expanding, intracranial, nitinol stent specifically designed for intracranial vessel stenosis (**Fig. 16**). It is produced by the same company that constructs the Neuroform stent and is a reinforced modification[88] with greater radial force to aid in long-term vessel dilation. The Wingspan stent is used in conjunction with a semicompliant balloon, the Gateway (Boston Scientific Corporation, Natick, MA). The Gateway balloon is inflated by means of a manometer and is used to compress atherosclerotic plaque at sites of stenosis with minimal trauma to the vessel wall before stent deployment.

Results with the Wingspan stent were first published in 2005.[88] A series of 15 patients who had symptomatic intracranial atherosclerosis despite medical therapy underwent placement of the Wingspan stent in the following manner. First, plaque compression and vessel dilatation with the Gateway balloon were performed to 80% of the parent vessel diameter. The Wingspan stent was passed over a microwire and positioned at the site of stenosis. It was deployed in a manner similar to that of Neuroform stent deployment, as described previously. Mean stenosis at the time of procedure was 72%, and it was reduced to 38% after stenting; there were no associated adverse events with the procedure.[88] Patients were started on antiplatelet therapy before the procedure and continued for 2 months afterward.[88] An HDE approval was granted by the FDA in 2005 for the Wingspan stent for treatment of intracranial stenosis of 50% or greater.[89] The Wingspan Study, a larger trial, was published in 2007; 45 patients who had symptomatic intracranial stenosis of 50% or greater were enrolled, and 44 underwent successful stent deployment.[89] Baseline average stenosis was 74.9%, which was reduced to 31.9% after stent deployment and to 28% at 6 months. Restenosis of 50% or greater was 7.5% at 6 months[89] and 26.3% at 1 year.[90] The 6- and 12-month ipsilateral stroke rates were 7.4% and 9.3%, respectively.[89]

The National Institutes of Health (NIH) Registry Wingspan study examined use of the Wingspan stent in symptomatic patients who had stenoses of 70% to 99%.[91] Zaidat and colleagues[91] compared their results with those of the Warfarin Aspirin Symptomatic Intracranial Disease (WASID) trial[84] in an attempt to analyze whether intracranial angioplasty and stenting improve the rates of yearly ischemic events when compared with maximal medical therapy. A total of 129 patients were enrolled, and 96.7% underwent successful stenting procedures. The mean prestent stenosis was 82% compared with 20% after stenting. Fifty-two patients underwent angiography at an average of 4.8 months, revealing a mean stenosis of 28%. Twenty-five percent of patients, however, were found to have 50% or greater restenosis. The rate of any stroke in 30 days, death in 30 days, and ipsilateral stroke later than 30 days from intervention was 14%.[91] When these patients were compared with a similar cohort from the WASID trial, the researchers found the event rates to diverge after 3 months, with fewer ischemic events occurring in the stented patients. The researchers concluded that a randomized trial between maximal medical therapy and angioplasty or stenting is needed.[91] The Stenting and Aggressive Medical Management for Preventing Recurrent Stroke in Intracranial Stenosis (SAMMPRIS) trial is planned[90] and plans to attempt to answer the question as to whether medical therapy or percutaneous angioplasty and stenting is the better treatment for symptomatic intracranial arterial stenosis to prevent recurrent ischemic events.

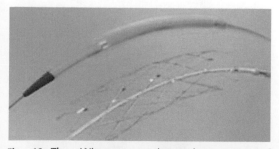

Fig. 16. The Wingspan endovascular stent and Gateway balloon. (*Courtesy of* Boston Scientific Corporation, Inc., Boston, MA; with permission.)

Authors' Management Strategy

Patients failing maximal medical therapy with angiographically proved intracranial large vessel stenosis of 50% to 99% are offered intracranial percutaneous angioplasty and stenting at the authors' institution. These procedures, as discussed elsewhere in this article, are performed under general anesthesia with neurophysiologic monitoring. The patients are placed on Plavix for 7 days before the procedure. In urgent circumstances, the authors may load the patient at the time of the procedure with 600 mg. After the procedure, the patient is to remain on aspirin indefinitely and on Plavix for 6 to 12 weeks. Once vascular access is achieved with a 7-French sheath, heparin is given (70 U/kg) to achieve an ACT two to three times that of baseline. MAP goals throughout the case are 80 to 90 mm Hg. Because

blood pressure frequently drops with anesthetic induction, vigilance is needed to support the patient's pressure and avoid possible tissue ischemia distal to a severe stenosis. DSA is performed with a 6-French Envoy guide catheter to localize the intracranial stenosis. A roadmap is created in two planes, a microwire is passed beyond the stenosis, and the Gateway balloon is sized to approximately 80% of the parent vessel diameter. The balloon is passed over the microwire to the site of stenosis. Filled with 30% contrast, it is slowly inflated with a manometer to a pressure between its rated nominal and bursting pressures and then deflated. DSA of the stenosis is performed to evaluate the extent of improvement after angioplasty. The balloon is removed, and the stent delivery device is passed over the wire and into position across the stenosis. It is

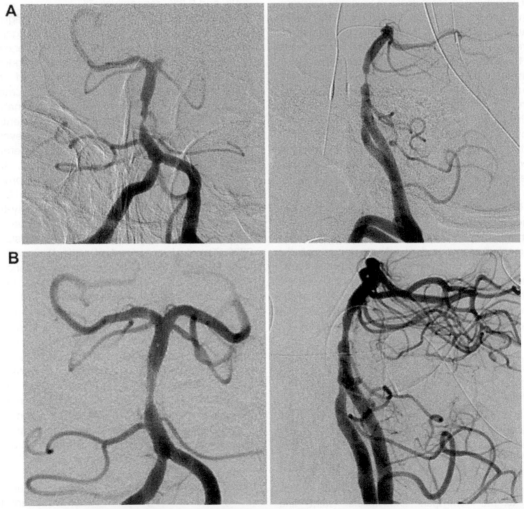

Fig. 17. (A) Digital subtraction angiogram shows severe basilar stenosis. (B) After Gateway balloon angioplasty and Wingspan stent (Boston Scientific, Fremont, CA) deployment. AP, anteroposterior.

deployed in the same manner as the Neuroform stent described previously. After deployment, DSA of the stenosis is performed to evaluate the effectiveness of the procedure (**Fig. 17**). Ideally, the stent is positioned to extend 3 mm on either side of the stenosis. Low-magnification intracranial DSA through the vessel of interest should be performed at the beginning and end of the procedure. The before and after runs are compared to ensure that all distal vessels remain patent and that the capillary and venous phases are unchanged.

SUMMARY

This article has examined the various techniques and devices involved in neuroendovascular procedures used to treat cerebral aneurysms, cerebral AVMs, acute cerebral ischemia, and symptomatic intracranial stenosis. The ability to access cerebral aneurysms is highly dependent on microwire and microcatheter technology to be able to "drive" the wire and catheter to the site of pathologic findings. The use of endovascular stents and improvements in coil technology have increased the number of aneurysms we are able to treat safely. Improvements in catheter and embolic agent technology have allowed us to treat AVMs once thought untreatable. Acute stroke intervention is now a reality thanks to the ability to deliver intra-arterial chemical agents and the advent of mechanical embolectomy devices. Additionally, patients who have intracranial stenosis now have new treatment options when medical therapy fails. As neuroendovascular technology continues to improve, so should our ability to treat patients who have complex cerebrovascular disorders more safely and effectively.

REFERENCES

1. Dawborn RHM. The starvation operation for malignancy in the external carotid area. JAMA 1904;17: 292–5.
2. Brooks B. The treatment of traumatic arteriovenous fistula. Southampt Med J 1930;23:100–16.
3. Lang ER, Bucy PC. Treatment of carotid-cavernous fistula by muscle embolization alone: the Brook's method. J Neurosurg 1965;22:387–92.
4. Luessenhop AJ, Spence WT. Artificial embolization of cerebral arteries; report of use in a case of arteriovenous malformations. JAMA 1960;172(11):1153–5.
5. Serbinenko FA. Balloon occlusion of cavernous portion of the carotid artery as a method of treating carotid-cavernous fistulae. Zh Vopr Neirokhir Im N N Burdenko 1971;6:3–9.
6. Debrun G, Lacour P, Caron JP, et al. Inflatable and released balloon technique experimentation in dog—application in man. Neuroradiology 1975;9: 267–71.
7. Spies JB, Berlin L. Complication of femoral artery puncture. AJR Am J Roentgenol 1998;170:9–11.
8. Seldinger SI. Catheter replacement of the needle in percutaneous arteriography; a new technique. Acta radiol 1953;39(5):368–76.
9. Turi ZG. Optimal femoral access prevents complications. Cardiac Interventions Today 2008;35–8.
10. Dandy WE. Intracranial aneurysms in the internal carotid artery. Ann Surg 1938;107:654–9.
11. Dandy WE. Intracranial arterial aneurysms of the carotid canal. Diagnosis and treatment. Arch Surg 1942;45:335–50.
12. Gallagher JP. The closure of intracranial aneurysms by pilojection. In: Fields WS, Sahs AL, editors. Intracranial aneurysms and subarachnoid hemorrhage. Springfield (IL): Charles C. Thomas; 1965. p. 357–71.
13. Mullan S, Raimondi AJ, Dobben G, et al. Electrically induced thrombosis in intracranial aneurysms. J Neurosurg 1965;22:539–47.
14. Mullan S, Reyes C, Dawley J. Stereotactic copper electric thrombosis of intracranial aneurysms. Prog Neurol Surg 1969;3:193–211.
15. Alskne JF, Fingerhurt AG, Rand RW. Magnetically controlled metallic thrombosis of intracranial aneurysms. Surgery 1966;60:212–8.
16. Alskne JF, Fingerhurt AG, Rand RW. Magnetic probe for the stereotactic thrombosis of intracranial aneurysms. J Neurol Neurosurg Psychiatr 1967;30: 159–62.
17. Debrun G, Fox A, Drake C, et al. Giant unclipped aneurysms: treatment with detachable balloons. AJNR Am J Neuroradiol 1981;2:167–73.
18. Guglielmi G, Viñuela F, Sepetka I, et al. Electrothrombosis of saccular aneurysms via endovascular approach. Part 1: electrochemical basis, technique, and experimental results. J Neurosurg 1991;75(1): 1–7.
19. Guglielmi G, Viñuela F, Dion J, et al. Electrothrombosis of saccular aneurysms via endovascular approach. Part 2: preliminary clinical experience. J Neurosurg 1991;75(1):8–14.
20. Prestigiacomo CJ. Surgical endovascular neuroradiology in the 21st century: what lies ahead? Neurosurgery 2006;59(5 Suppl 3):S48–55.
21. Cognard C, Weill A, Spelle L, et al. Long-term angiographic follow-up of 169 intracranial berry aneurysms occluded with detachable coils. Radiology 1999;212:348–56.
22. Raymond J, Guilbert F, Weill A, et al. Long-term angiographic recurrence after selective endovascular treatment of aneurysms with detachable coils. Stroke 2003;34:1398–403.

23. Veznedaroglu E, Koebbe C, Siddiqui A, et al. Initial experience with bioactive Cerecyte detachable coils: impact on reducing recurrence rate. Neurosurgery 2008;62(4):799–805.

24. Fiorella D, Albuquerque FC, McDougall CG. Durability of aneurysm embolization with matrix detachable coils. Neurosurgery 2006;58:51–9.

25. Murayama Y, Tateshima S, Gonzalez NR, et al. Matrix and bioabsorbable polymeric coils accelerate healing of intracranial aneurysms: long-term experimental study. Stroke 2003;34:2031–7.

26. Murayama Y, Vinuela F, Tateshima S, et al. Bioabsorbable polymeric material coils for embolization of intracranial aneurysms: a preliminary experimental study. J Neurosurg 2001;94:454–63.

27. Niimi Y, Song J, Madrid M, et al. Endosaccular treatment of intracranial aneurysms using matrix coils: early experience and midterm follow-up. Stroke 2006;37:1028–32.

28. Cloft HJ. HydroCoil for Endovascular Aneurysm Occlusion (HEAL) study: periprocedural results. AJNR Am J Neuroradiol 2006;27:289–92.

29. Vallée JN, Pierot L, Bonafé A, et al. Endovascular treatment of intracranial wide-necked aneurysms using three-dimensional coils: predictors of immediate anatomic and clinical results. AJNR Am J Neuroradiol 2004;25:298–306.

30. Fernandez Zubillaga A, Guglielmi G, Viñuela F, et al. Endovascular occlusion of intracranial aneurysms with electrically detachable coils: correlation of aneurysm neck size and treatment results. AJNR Am J Neuroradiol 1994;15:815–20.

31. Moret J, Cognard C, Weill A, et al. The "remodelling technique" in the treatment of wide neck intracranial aneurysms. Intervent Neuroradiol 1997;3: 21–35.

32. DeBrun GM, Aletich VA, Kehrli P, et al. Selection of cerebral aneurysms for treatment using Guglielmi detachable coils: the preliminary University of Illinois at Chicago experience. Neurosurgery 1998;43: 1281–95.

33. Lefkowitz MA, Gobin YP, Akiba Y, et al. Balloon-assisted Guglielmi detachable coiling of wide-necked aneurysms: part II. Clinical results. Neurosurgery 1999;45:531–8.

34. Sluzewski M, Rooij WJV, Beute GN, et al. Balloon-assisted coil embolization of intracranial aneurysms: incidence, complications, and angiography results. J Neurosurg 2006;105(3):396–9.

35. Pelz DM, Lownie SP, Fox AJ. Thromboembolic events associated with the treatment of cerebral aneurysms with Guglielmi detachable coils. AJNR Am J Neuroradiol 1998;19:1541–7.

36. Soeda A, Sakia H, Sakai H, et al. Thromboembolic events associated with Guglielmi detachable coil embolization of asymptomatic cerebral aneurysms: evaluation of 66 consecutive cases with the use of diffusion-weighted MRI imaging. AJNR Am J Neuroradiol 2003;24:127–32 [My paper].

37. Phatouros CC, Halbach VV, Malek AM, et al. Simultaneous subarachnoid hemorrhage and carotid-cavernous sinus fistula after rupture of paraclinoid aneurysms during balloon-assisted coil embolization. AJNR Am J Neuroradiol 1999;20:1100–2.

38. Biondi A, Janardhan V, Katz J, et al. Neuroform stent-assisted coil embolization of wide-necked intracranial aneurysms: strategies in stent deployment and midterm follow-up. Neurosurgery 2007; 61(3):460–9.

39. Benitez RP, Silva MT, Klem J, et al. Endovascular occlusion of wide-necked aneurysms with a new intracranial microstent (Neuroform) and detachable coils. Neurosurgery 2004;54(6):1359–67.

40. Mocco J, Snyder KV, Albuquerque FC, et al. Treatment of intracranial aneurysms with the Enterprise stent: a multicenter registry. J Neurosurg 2008;110: 35–9.

41. Mawad ME, Cekirge S, Ciceri E, et al. Endovascular treatment of giant and large intracranial aneurysms by using a combination of stent placement and liquid polymer injection. J Neurosurg 2002;96: 474–82.

42. Doppman JL, DiChiro G, Ommaya AK. Percutaneous embolization of spinal cord arteriovenous malformations. J Neurosurg 1971;34:48–54.

43. Kerber C. Balloon catheter with a calibrated leak. A new system for superselective angiography and occlusion catheter technology. Radiology 1976; 120:547–50.

44. Jafar JJ, Davis AJ, Berenstein A, et al. The effect of embolization with n-butylcyanoacrylate prior to surgical resection of cerebral arteriovenous malformations. J Neuorosurg 1993;78(1):60–9.

45. DeMeritt JS, Pile-Spellman J, Moohan N, et al. Outcome analysis of preoperative embolization with n-butylcyanoacrylate in cerebral arteriovenous malformations. AJNR Am J Neuroradiol 1997;16: 1801–7.

46. Fiorella D, Albuquerque FC, McDougall CG, et al. The role of neuroendovascular therapy for the treatment of brain arteriovenous malformations. Neurosurgery 2006;59(5 Suppl 3):S163–77.

47. Frizzel RT, Fisher WS 3rd. Cure, morbidity, and mortality associated with embolization of brain arteriovenous malformations: a review of 1246 patients in 32 series over a 35-year period. Neurosurgery 1995;37(6):1031–9.

48. Gobin YP, Laurent A, Merienne L, et al. Treatment of brain arteriovenous malformations by embolization and radiosurgery. J Neurosurg 1996;85(1): 19–28.

49. Valavanis A, Yasargil MG. The endovascular treatment of brain arteriovenous malformation. Adv Tech Stand Neurosurg 1998;24:131–214.

50. Yu SCH, Chan MSY, Lam JMK, et al. Complete obliteration of intracranial arteriovenous malformations with endovascular cyanoacrylate embolization: initial success and rate of permanent cure. AJNR Am J Neuroradiol 2004;25(7):1139–43.

51. Al-Yamany M, Terbrugge KG, Willinsky R. Palliative embolization of brain arteriovenous malformations presenting with progressive neurological deficit. Intervent Neuroradiol 2000;6:177–83.

52. Meisel HJ, Mansmann U, Alvarez H, et al. Effect of partial targeted n-butyl-cyano-acrylate embolization in brain AVM. Acta Neurochir (Wein) 2002;144(9):879–87.

53. Miyomoto S, Hashimoto N, Nagata I, et al. Posttreatment sequelae of palliatively treated cerebral arteriovenous malformations. Neurosurgery 2000;46(3):589–94.

54. Kwon OK, Han DH, Han MH, et al. Palliatively treated cerebral arteriovenous malformations: follow-up results. J Clin Neurosci 2000;7(Suppl 1):69–72.

55. Sorimachi T, Koike T, Takeuchi S, et al. Embolization of cerebral arteriovenous malformations achieved with polyvinyl alcohol particles: angiographic reappearance and complications. AJNR Am J Neuroradiol 1999;20:1323–8.

56. Mathis JA, Barr JD, Horton JA, et al. The efficacy of particulate embolization combined with stereotactic radiosurgery for treatment for large arteriovenous malformations of the brain. AJNR Am J Neuroradiol 1995;16:299–306.

57. Pelz DM, Fox AJ, Vinuela F, et al. Preoperative embolization of brain AVMs with isobutyl-2-cyanoacrylate. AJNR Am J Neuroradiol 1988;9(4):757–64.

58. Taki W, Yonekawa Y, Iwata H, et al. A new liquid material for embolization of arteriovenous malformations. AJNR Am J Neuroradiol 1990;11:163–8.

59. Murayama Y, Vinuela F, Ulhoa A, et al. Nonadhesive liquid embolic agent for cerebral arteriovenous malformations: preliminary histopathological studies in swine rete mirabile. Neurosurgery 1998;43:1164–75.

60. Jahan R, Murayama Y, Gobin YP, et al. Embolization of arteriovenous malformations with Onyx: clinicopathological experience in 23 patients. Neurosurgery 2001;48:984–97.

61. Yakes WF, Rossi P, Odink H. Arteriovenous malformations management. How I do it. Cardiovasc Intervent Radiol 1996;19:65–71.

62. Rosamond W, Flegal K, Furie K, et al. Heart disease and stroke statistics 2008 update: a report from the American Heart Association Statistics Committee and Stroke Statistics Subcommittee. Circulation 2008;117:e25–146.

63. Fieschi C, Argentino C, Lenzi GL, et al. Clinical and instrumental evaluation of patients with ischemic stroke within the first six hours. J Neurosurg Sci 1989;91:311–22.

64. del Zoppo GJ, Poeck K, Pessin MS, et al. Recombinant tissue plasminogen activator in acute thrombotic and embolic stroke. Ann Neurol 1992;32:78–86.

65. Furlan AJ. Natural history of atherothromboembolic occlusion of cerebral arteries: carotid versus vertebrobasilar territories. In: Hacke W, del Zoppo GJ, Hirschberg M, editors. Thrombolytic therapy in acute ischemic stroke. New York: Springer-Verlag; 1991. p. 71–6.

66. The National Institute of Neurological Disorders and Stroke rt-PA Stroke Study Group. Tissue plasminogen activator for acute ischemic stroke. N Engl J Med 1995;333(24):1581–7.

67. del Zoppo GJ, Higashida RT, Furlan AJ, et al. PROACT: a phase II randomized trial of recombinant prourokinase by direct arterial delivery in acute middle cerebral artery stroke. Stroke 1998;29:4–11.

68. Furlan AJ, Higashida RT, Wechsler L, et al. Intraarterial prourokinase for acute ischemic stroke: the PROACT II study: a randomized controlled trial. JAMA 1999;282(21):2003–11.

69. ASITN, ASNR Stroke Task Force, SCIVR. Emergency interventional stroke therapy: a statement from the American Society of Interventional Therapeutic Neuroradiology, Stroke Task Force of the American Society of Neuroradiology, and the Society of Cardiovascular and Interventional Radiology. AJNR Am J Neuroradiol 2001;22:54.

70. Lewandowski CA, Frankel M, Tomsick TA, et al. Combined intravenous and intra-arterial r-TPA versus intra-arterial therapy of acute ischemic stroke: Emergency Management of Stroke (EMS) bridging trial. Stroke 1999;30:2598–605.

71. The IMS Study Investigators. Combined intravenous and intra-arterial recanalization for acute ischemic stroke: the Interventional Management of Stroke study. Stroke 2004;35:904–11.

72. Gobin YP, Starkman S, Duckwiler GR, et al. MERCI 1: a phase 1 study of mechanical embolus removal in cerebral ischemia. Stroke 2004;35:2848–54.

73. Smith WS, Sung G, Starkman S, et al. Safety and efficacy of mechanical embolectomy in acute ischemic stroke. Results of the MERCI trial. Stroke 2005;36:1432–40.

74. Smith WS. Safety of mechanical thrombectomy and intravenous tissue plasminogen activator in acute ischemic stroke. Results of the multi Mechanical Embolus Removal in Cerebral Ischemia (MERCI) trial, part I. AJNR Am J Neuroradiol 2006;27:1177–82.

75. Flint AC, Duckwiler GR, Budzik RF, et al. Mechanical thrombectomy of intracranial internal carotid occlusion. Pooled results of the MERCI and Multi MERCI Part I trials. Stroke 2007;38:1274–80.

76. Smith WS, Sung G, Saver J, et al. Mechanical thrombectomy for acute ischemic stroke: final results of the Multi MERCI trial. Stroke 2008;39:1205–12.

77. Available at: http://www.concentric-medical.com/webpage.php?ln_id=60. Accessed January 10, 2009.

78. Available at: http://www.penumbrainc.com/products/penumbra-system. Accessed January 10, 2009.

79. Bose A, Henkes H, Alfke K, et al. The Penumbra System: a mechanical device for the treatment of acute stroke due to thromboembolism. AJNR Am J Neuroradiol 2008;29:1409–13.

80. Sacco RL, Kargman DE, Gu Q, et al. Race-ethnicity and determinants of intracranial atherosclerotic cerebral infarction: The Northern Manhattan Stroke Study. Stroke 1995;26:14–20.

81. Chimowitz MI, Kokkinos J, Strong J, et al. The Warfarin-Aspirin Symptomatic Intracranial Disease Study. Neurology 1995;45:1488–93.

82. The Warfarin-Aspirin Symptomatic Intracranial Disease (WASID) Study Group. Prognosis of patients with symptomatic vertebral or basilar artery stenosis. Stroke 1998;29:1389–92.

83. Thijs VN, Albers GW. Symptomatic intracranial atherosclerosis: outcome of patients who fail antithrombotic therapy. Neurology 2000;55:490–7.

84. Chimowitz MI, Lynn MJ, Howlett-Smith H, et al, for the Warfarin-Aspirin Symptomatic Intracranial Disease Trial Investigators. Comparison of warfarin and aspirin for symptomatic intracranial arterial stenosis. N Engl J Med 2005;352:1305–16.

85. Kasner SE, Chimowitz MI, Lynn MJ, et al, for the Warfarin Aspirin Symptomatic Intracranial Disease (WASID) Trial Investigators. Predictors of ischemic stroke in the territory of a symptomatic intracranial arterial stenosis. Circulation 2006;113:555–63.

86. Mazighi M, Tanasescu R, Ducrocq X, et al. Prospective study of symptomatic atherothrombotic intracranial stenoses: the GESICA study. Neurology 2006;1187–91.

87. The SSYLVIA Study Investigators. Stenting of Symptomatic Atherosclerotic Lesions in the Vertebral or Intracranial Arteries (SSYLVIA): study results. Stroke 2004;35:1388–92.

88. Henkes H, Miloslavski E, Lowens S, et al. Treatment of intracranial atherosclerotic stenoses with balloon dilatation and self-expanding stent deployment (WingSpan). Neuroradiology 2005;47(3):222–8.

89. Bose A, Hartmann M, Henkes H, et al. A novel, self-expanding, nitinol stent in medically refractory intracranial atherosclerotic stenoses: the Wingspan study. Stroke 2007;38:1531–7.

90. Leung TW, Yu SCH, Lam WWM, et al. The NIH registry on use of the Wingspan stent for symptomatic 70-99% intracranial arterial stenosis. Neurology 2008;71(14):1125–35.

91. Zaidat OO, Klucznik R, Alexander MJ, et al. The NIH registry on use of the Wingspan stent for symptomatic 70-99% intracranial arterial stenosis. Neurology 2008;70(17):1518–24.

Percutaneous Vertebroplasty

Michael C. Hurley, MD[a,b], Rami Kaakaji, MD[b],
Guilherme Dabus, MD[a,b], Ali Shaibani, MD[a,b],
Mathew T. Walker, MD[b], Richard G. Fessler, MD[a],
Bernard R. Bendok, MD[a,b],*

KEYWORDS

- Vertebroplasty • Compression • Osteoporosis
- Kyphoplasty • Augmentation • Percutaneous

First performed in 1984 by Galibert and Deramond in the treatment of an aggressive vertebral hemangioma,[1] percutaneous vertebroplasty is a minimally invasive technique employing the injection of liquid polymethylmethacylate cement into a fractured vertebral body to relieve pain, reinforce the bone, and prevent further vertebral compression. The basic technique varies depending on the location, severity, and cause of the vertebral fracture. Successful practice requires careful patient selection, a sound understanding of the technique, and an ability to troubleshoot pitfalls. This article addresses each of these requirements in turn and then discusses the evidence supporting vertebroplasty and associated controversies.

The majority of vertebral fractures referred for vertebroplasty are secondary to vertebral insufficiency caused by osteoporosis. Osteoporosis afflicts 28 million people in the United States[2-4] and is responsible for approximately 750,000 spinal fractures per year.[5] Osteoporosis may be primary, as affects a third of white postmenopausal women, or secondary to the use of steroids and other medications, hyperthyroidism, chronic disease, renal impairment, and other conditions.[6,7] The consequences of vertebral compression fractures should not be underestimated: a retrospective study of the Medicare population in the United States found that the 7-year mortality rate for patients over 65 years of age who had vertebral compression fractures was almost double that of matched controls.[8-12]

Conventional management consists of a mix of analgesic medication, bed rest, orthotic braces, and physiotherapy.[13-16] The problems of opioid dependency and prolonged bed rest can result in a vicious cycle of physical deconditioning, poor nutrition, and increased risk of vertebral insufficiency.[17] Other risks include decubitus ulceration, nosocomial infection, deep venous thrombosis, and mood disorder, all of which prolong the recovery period and result in a loss of independence.[18,19] Despite these concerns, most patients improve within 2 months of a symptomatic compression fracture.[20] Patients who have osteoporosis are at increased risk of subsequent vertebral and non-vertebral fractures[21] and should commence appropriate regimens to strengthen the bone matrix, including smoking cessation, increased dietary intake of calcium and vitamin D, physiotherapy, and use of bisphosphonates, calcitonin, or estrogen agonists as appropriate.[22]

PATIENT SELECTION AND WORK-UP
Indications

The primary goal of vertebroplasty is to provide relief of distressing and debilitating pain caused by vertebral compression fractures after a failure of conservative therapy, traditionally defined as a lack of improvement after 4 to 6 weeks. Some

a Department of Neurosurgery, Northwestern University Feinberg School of Medicine, 676 North St. Clair Street Suite 2210, Chicago, IL 60611, USA
b Division of Neuroradiology, Department of Radiology, Northwestern University Feinberg School of Medicine, 676 North St. Clair Street Suite 800, Chicago, IL 60611, USA
* Corresponding author.
E-mail address: bbendok@nmff.org (B.R. Bendok).

Neurosurg Clin N Am 20 (2009) 341–359
doi:10.1016/j.nec.2009.03.001
1042-3680/09/$ – see front matter © 2009 Elsevier Inc. All rights reserved.

practitioners now recommend earlier intervention in selected cases to avoid the risks of general deconditioning and iatrogenic complications mentioned previously. Earlier treatment also may give a greater chance of height restoration, although the merits of this claim are controversial, as discussed later.

The operator must be satisfied that there is a significant symptomatic contribution from the vertebral fracture(s) considered for treatment. Difficulties in assessment frequently arise in the typical elderly patient who has advanced degenerative spondylosis or in cases with multiple compression fractures of various ages. Positive clinical indicators of an acute insufficiency compression injury that will respond well to vertebroplasty include a report of a sudden, recent onset of pain or a specific trigger such as a minor trauma. Even if the patient is a good historian, back pain often localizes the source poorly,[23] and although it is reassuring if the examination elicits midline tenderness within one to two levels of the fractured vertebra, the absence of this finding should not obviate treatment.[24] A formal 10-point or visual analog baseline pain score,[25] ideally supplemented by a disability assessment, should be recorded so that a future assessment of response to treatment can be made. The examination should document any radiculopathy or motor or sensory deficits before treatment.

Although, non-osteoporotic causes of vertebral fractures, such as trauma and neoplasia (metastases, myeloma, lymphoma, hemangioma),

usually are diagnosed before presentation for vertebroplasty, a suspected neoplasm may be biopsied at the time of treatment.[26,27] Vertebroplasty also can be combined with radiofrequency ablation in a single sitting,[28,29] as described later.

Imaging

Standard standing anteroposterior (AP) and lateral spine radiographs should confirm the presence of a fracture but are unreliable both in determining the age of the lesion without a recent comparison and in assessing fracture stability (eg, as in a simple wedge versus a burst fracture).[30]

MR T2-weighted short-tau inversion recovery (STIR) sequences are exquisitely sensitive to T2-hyperintense vertebral edema (**Fig. 1**), the presence of which suggests an acute or progressive fracture that is more likely to respond to vertebroplasty.[31] Patients without compressive deformity but with vertebral edema may have non-deforming microfractures and also be candidates for vertebroplasty.[32] Fluid-filled fracture clefts are best depicted on T2-STIR MRI, although their association with ongoing pain is less robust than that of the less common gas-filled cleft. Enhancement after gadolinium injection is seen commonly in insufficiency fractures and in this context may indicate a symptomatic lesion more likely to respond to treatment.[33] Enhancement also should lead to careful scrutiny for evidence of neoplasia (eg, disproportionate enhancement or lesions in the posterior elements or paravertebral region).

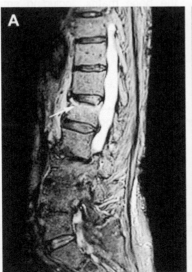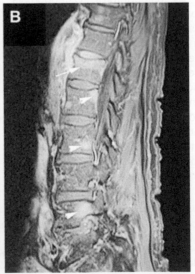

Fig. 1. MR features of recent compression fractures. (*A*) Edema (*arrow*) around an L1 superior endplate insufficiency fracture in an elderly woman who has prominent degenerative changes. (*B*) Contrast enhancement in an insufficiency fracture (*arrow*) compared with enhancing metastatic disease (*arrowheads*).

Osteomyelitis, an absolute contraindication to vertebroplasty, characteristically involves the vertebral endplate, although an uncommon pattern of septic vertebral emboli mimicking metastases has been described.[34] MRI is also an excellent means of assessing the spinal canal, particularly in cases of tumor extension, which is less obvious on CT. An endplate cortical defect on MRI, fluid in the adjacent disc, and lack of a vertebral cleft increase the risk of extravasation into the disc space.[35]

CT demonstrates mineralized bone exquisitely and has higher spatial resolution than standard MR sequences. Gas-filled fracture clefts that are associated with ongoing pain are more readily appreciated on CT. CT is less reliable in establishing the age of a fracture, because acute compaction of the trabecular framework can simulate a chronic osteoblastic process. Defects in the posterior vertebral wall or displaced fragments are well demonstrated. The pedicular size also can be better assessed, helping the choice of needle size and approach.

Bone scintigraphy helps to identify "active," healing lesions with osteoblastic activity. Like MRI, bone scintigraphy also predicts a symptomatic response to vertebroplasty[36] and may be more reliable in older fractures (> 3 or 4 months).[37] In the authors' experience, however, a bone scan usually is unnecessary if an MRI has been performed.

PROCEDURE AND TECHNIQUE
Preprocedure Work-Up

Although most patients tolerate the procedure under moderate sedation, patients who have respiratory difficulty and those who may not tolerate the prone position because of their habitus or discomfort should be assessed by the anesthesiology service for the use of monitored anesthesia care or general anesthesia.[38,39] These patients are prone to acute deterioration, with even small pulmonary emboli (cement, air, or marrow) causing critical decompensation.

Any history of recent infection should be sought, and, if the history is positive, the patient should receive a full course of antibiotic treatment before the procedure with documented eradication of the offending organism. All patients receive a preoperative intravenous antibiotic, cefazolin (2 g), clindamycin (900 mg) or vancomycin (1 g), depending on any history of adverse reactions. Coagulopathy is a relative contraindication to vertebroplasty, and an international normalized ratio (INR) and partial thromboplastin time (PTT) should be assessed. Cut-off levels vary around an INR of 1.4 and PTT of 50 seconds. Significant coagulopathy may require correction with vitamin K or fresh-frozen plasma.

The patient's imaging should be reviewed again before the procedure, and any potential difficulty in identifying the treatment level fluoroscopically should be anticipated (eg, in cases with transitional vertebral or rib anatomy). Previous spinal instrumentation and vertebral deformities can be used as landmarks. The authors routinely count up from L5 and down from T1 to confirm the appropriate level. It also should be possible to determine the optimal vertebroplasty needle size and approach (transpedicular or parapedicular and unilateral versus bilateral pedicles).

Informed consent must highlight the rationale (fracture augmentation leading to pain relief), benefits (expedited pain relief and mobilization), risks (particularly cord or radicular compromise and pulmonary embolism), and alternatives (conservative treatment). The possibility that the procedure will provide a disappointing degree of pain relief because of the degree of comorbid disease should be evaluated and explained.

Procedural Equipment

A biplane fluoroscopy unit is preferable for needle navigation and monitoring of cement penetration. A single-plane unit can be used but adds significantly to the procedure time, particularly with older units, and can lead to a compromise in the surveillance for cement migration.

A 22-gauge spinal needle is used to infiltrate 1% to 2% lidocaine down to the periosteum. A T-extension tube is indispensable to enable manipulation of the needle under the image intensifier while injecting.

When selecting a vertebroplasty needle (**Fig. 2**), larger gauges and shorter lengths generate less resistance during cement injection, resulting in better feedback and control. Lumbar pedicles should accommodate an 11-gauge needle, and thoracic pedicles should accommodate a 13-gauge needle. Smaller pedicles in the upper thoracic and cervical spine may require a 15-gauge needle, also useful for treatment of a vertebra plana. Lengths of 10 cm are sufficient in most cases; longer 15-cm needles are more unwieldy but are necessary in obese patients. Most needles have a large plastic handle for rotation and withdrawal that can obscure the needle tip if fluoroscopy is angled down the barrel of the needle. These handles also can impinge on each other when multiple levels are accessed simultaneously. Standard needle tips are diamond-shaped, giving better initial

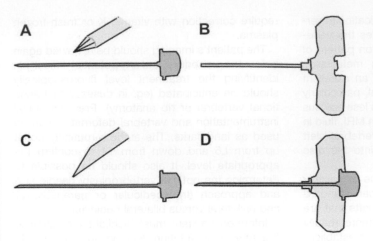

Fig. 2. Typical vertebroplasty needles. The cutting edge is located on the tip of the trochar with the commonly used (A) diamond tip and (C) bevelled tip illustrated. (B) The outer cannula has a blunt and flush tip. Note the large handle to assist cannula retraction. (D) The trochar should lock securely into position when loaded into the outer cannula.

purchase, or beveled, offering an added degree of navigability.

Dedicated cement injectors are designed to allow the operator to stand further from the image intensifier and to avoid exposure to large radiation doses (**Fig. 3**). Some operators prefer to inject through the needle with multiple 1-mL syringes that are preloaded with cement, allowing better control but larger radiation exposure.

A needle driver (forceps) is useful as a radiopaque marker when mapping out the approach and for manipulating the needle under continuous fluoroscopy while avoiding direct irradiation to the operator's hand.

Most available cements are polymethylmethacrylate that is provided as a powder polymer and liquid monomer that gradually set after being vigorously mixed. Sterile barium, tantalum, or zirconium dioxide is mixed into the cement to provide contrast. Most operators no longer consider the addition of an antibiotic, such as tobramycin, to the cement mixture necessary.

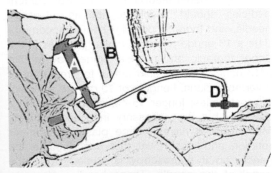

Fig. 3. Using a (A) cement injector and (C) connecting tube attached to the (D) vertebroplasty needle, the operator can stand behind a (B) lead screen and reduce their radiation exposure.

A mallet is provided to tap the needle through bone but may not be necessary in cases of severe osteoporosis.

A trephinated biopsy can be performed through the vertebroplasty needle before injecting cement. A 14-gauge biopsy needle works well through an 11-gauge vertebroplasty needle.

Procedure

Patient positioning

Patients are placed prone on the fluoroscopy table with supplemental oxygen administered via nasal cannula and continuous respiratory and cardiac monitoring. A bolster may be placed under the patient's abdomen to increase comfort. Moderate sedation is administered by boluses of a benzodiazepine and opiate; the authors usually start with midazolam (2 mg) and fentanyl (50 μg), depending on respiratory baseline. Spot images of the spine can be recorded to document the pertinent anatomy used to identify the correct level.

Optimizing tube angulation

The x-ray tube angulation is corrected for the patient's positioning on the table. Close attention must be made to ensure the B-tube/lateral gives a true lateral view of the vertebra being treated and should be aimed to superimpose the pedicles, ribs, and transverse processes. The vertebral endplate will not align if there is an asymmetrical compression deformity. The A-tube either is angled to get a true AP view of the vertebral body or is angled down the barrel of the pedicle being used for access. The former approach allows a clearer assessment of the amount of needle angulation required to reach the midline vertebral body, whereas the latter gives a better definition of the critical anatomic landmark comprising the medial pedicular cortex (the AP view can be resumed after the needle has cleared the pedicle and entered the posterior vertebral body).

Local anesthesia

It is important to infiltrate local anesthetic down to the periosteum over the pedicle. If multiple pedicles are to be traversed, note that the recommended maximum adult dose of lidocaine is 300 mg (30 cc of 1% or 15 cc of 2%) in a 90-minute period. A standard 22-gauge 3.5-inch spinal needle usually will reach the bony entry site (usually the crotch formed by the transverse process and lamina).

Vertebroplasty needle placement

The cutaneous entry puncture site and needle trajectory must be optimized to avoid complications (**Fig. 4**). A 1-cm incision is made in the skin at the puncture site. When the operator is looking down the barrel of the pedicle on the A-plane and is using a needle driver to avoid exposure of the operator's hands, the needle is directed straight down the line of the fluoroscopic beam ("dotting" the needle) and onto the upper-outer part of the oval outline of the pedicle (**Fig. 5**). The width of the pedicle then can be used maximally to gain extra angulation toward the midline. The

A-plane is rotated slightly to avoid obscuring the needle tip by the shaft and handle. Before advancing the needle, the lateral view is used to ensure correct alignment of the needle along the pedicle in the sagittal plane. The needle is advanced at first by multiple small taps with the mallet, and the force required to advance the needle can be judged by observing its progress with simultaneous fluoroscopy on the lateral view, which, unlike the A-plane, can be collimated to avoid direct exposure of the operator's hands. The needle is advanced in small increments with subsequent assessment on both projections to ensure safe positioning. When the needle gains purchase within the bone, the needle driver is no longer needed. If a beveled needle is used, the tip will tend to migrate away from the open face of the bevel, which can be rotated to help guide the tip to the desired location. After the posterior body is entered, there is no longer a risk of breaching the medial pedicle and canal; therefore the operator can concentrate on landing the tip in the optimal part of the vertebral body. When a single needle is used, best results are achieved with a tip placement in the midline, at the junction of the mid and anterior thirds and above or below the equator (to avoid the basivertebral venous

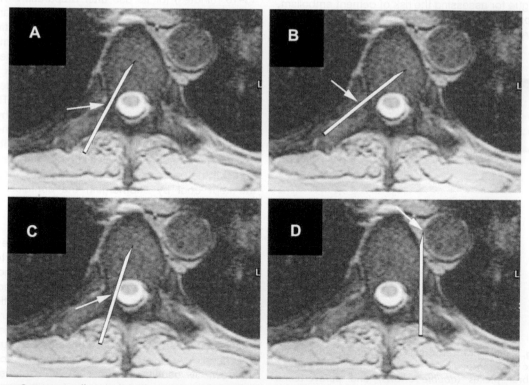

Fig. 4. Correct needle access into a thoracic vertebra via the (*A*) pedicular and (*B*) costo-transverse routes. (*C*) Aberrant entry breaching the right canal and thecal sac. (*D*) Lateral passage causing an aortic injury.

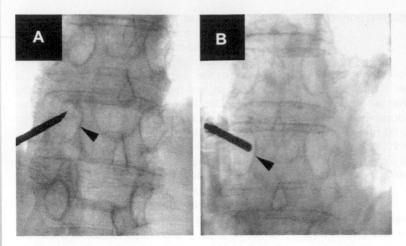

Fig. 5. (*A*) The needle is lined up for skin incision. (*B*) The needle is advanced to the posterior vertebral body. Note non-transgression of the medial pedicular cortex (*arrowhead* in *A* and *B*).

plexus). If a bipedicular technique is used, the needles are placed with the tips on either side of the midline. If there is a fracture cleft, some operators recommend targeting this cleft directly, as discussed later. When the trochar is removed, blood can ooze briskly through the needle, depending on the basivertebral venous pressure, but the oozing should subside rapidly. The trochar should be left in the needle during cement preparation to avoid significant blood loss. Iodinated contrast venography (**Fig. 6**) previously was in vogue for assessing the risk of cement embolism. Most, however, consider this imaging an unnecessary step that can result in retained vertebral

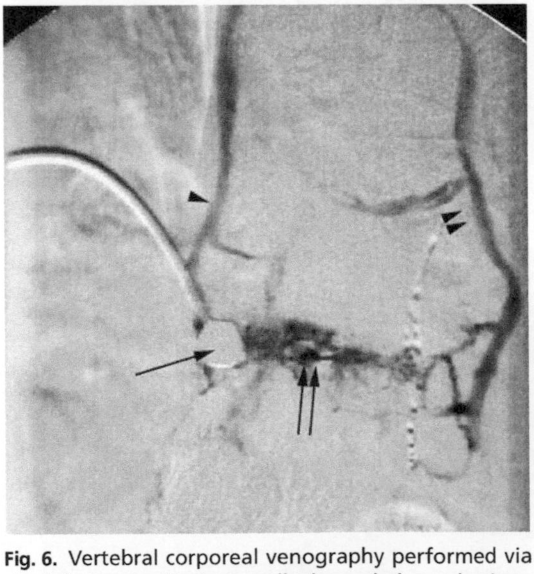

contrast obscuring the working views. If multiple levels are to be treated, the operator either can treat one at a time or can place the needles at multiple levels before cement injection. The latter technique may be more efficient and allow two levels to be treated with the same cement preparation.

Cement preparation

The cement is prepared only after needle placement because of the limited window of time (5–10 minutes) for its use after preparation. The method of preparation varies with the brand used, and even very minor deviation in relative volumes of barium, polymer, and liquid monomer can result in significant differences in the cement viscosity. The cement is poured into the back of the injector syringe, the syringe driver is loaded, and the air is expelled from the system. The cement viscosity usually is satisfactory if, when dripped onto the table, the drips visibly hold their form before merging into a pool, similar to toothpaste. The cement sets faster at higher temperatures; if the operator is not ready to inject, it can be kept cool by submerging the container in pre-refrigerated saline.

Cement injection

The injector is connected via a connecting tube to the vertebroplasty needle, and cement is injected slowly under lateral fluoroscopic surveillance. The cement should be visible within the needle before it exits the tip, and the rate of injection should be adjusted to avoid a sudden discharge into the vertebra. Most of the resistance to injection is generated by the transit of cement through the needle. As the cement enters the vertebral marrow, it usually assumes a characteristic trabecular pattern that helps confirm its appropriate distribution. If cement does extend beyond

Fig. 6. Vertebral corporeal venography performed via the left transpedicular needle (*arrow*) shows basivertebral plexus (*double arrows*) and paravertebral drainage via the azygous (*double arrowheads*) and hemiazygous (*arrowhead*) veins.

the margin of the vertebral body, it will tend to form a more homogenous globule. Continuous fluoroscopy is mandatory during the entire injection, mainly with lateral surveillance supplemented by intermittent assessment of the AP view. Tip placement in a basivertebral vein characterized by washout of the radiodense cement by non-opacified blood flow, most often occurs at the beginning of the injection, and usually ceases after a pause to allow the injected cement to occlude the channel. The injection should be halted if cement migrates to the posterior quarter of the vertebral body, through the endplate into the disc space, or into the paravertebral space. Rotating the needle tip (if beveled) or withdrawing the needle a short distance may result in an altered passage of cement. Repeated encroachment on the posterior quarter of the vertebral body should lead to termination of cement injection through that needle. One should note that the midline posterior wall of the vertebra is a few millimeters more anterior than its outer edges because of its concave posterior curvature. The goal is to reinforce the anterior portion of the body and fill any fracture clefts; if this goal is achieved, no additional structural benefit is gained from trying to fill the remainder of the body with cement. If the cement becomes too viscous to inject before adequate filling of the vertebra, it usually is still possible to push it through the needle using the trochar.

Needle withdrawal

When withdrawing the needle, it is important not to draw a strand of cement back through the soft tissues, because when this strand hardens it can cause discomfort and increase the risk of infection. Rotating the needle several times at the completion of the injection helps detach the tip from the injected cement, and the needle should be closely observed under lateral fluoroscopy during withdrawal. In certain cases, such as a pedicular fracture, the operator may choose to perform additional pediculoplasty by injecting cement into the pedicle when withdrawing the needle. Extreme care is required, given the proximity to the canal, and only a tiny volume of cement is necessary. When the needle has been removed, hemostasis usually can be achieved by massaging the soft tissues around the puncture site and by a short period of manual compression. Spot images of the treated levels should be performed before transferring the patient off the table.

Postprocedure care

The patient is observed during supine bed rest for 2 hours and undergoes a check non-contrast CT through the treated level. State-of-the-art fluoroscopy units offer integrated cone-beam tomography, which may negate the need for a subsequent regular CT.[40] Patients are reassessed with a formal pain score to document their early response to the treatment before discharge. They can be followed up at 1 to 2 weeks for a final assessment before being discharged to their primary care physician.

Modified Techniques

Parapedicular approach

In the upper thoracic spine the pedicles are small and have a more perpendicular orientation back from the vertebral body, making it difficult to angle the needle toward the midline. A costotransverse approach allows greater angulation and maintains a safe distance between the needle and the canal/neural foramen (see **Fig. 4**). This approach is particularly helpful when the pedicle is poorly visualized because of a destructive lesion or patient habitus.

Curved needle

The advantages of using a curved-needle coaxial system are the ability to target selectively different segments of the vertebral body, such as fracture clefts, and more reliable penetration across the midline (**Fig. 7**).[41] If cement migrates in an unfavorable direction, the probe can be repositioned. Custom systems now are available comprising a 13-gauge blunt-tipped nitinol needle with a 95° angle that is delivered through a 10- or 11-gauge needle, which initially is advanced into the posterior aspect of the vertebral body.[42] Multiple passes of the needle may help create a communicating central vertebral cavity before cement injection.[43]

CT guidance

In rare cases, such as severe vertebra plana or bony destruction, the needle can be placed initially under CT control, and the patient then can be transferred to the fluoroscopy unit to undergo surveillance during the cement injection. This procedure is lengthy, requiring prolonged patient sedation, and taxes staff resources. Although the technique has been described,[44,45] the authors do not consider the CT-fluoroscopy technology currently available in most centers to provide adequate real-time surveillance of cement migration.

Cervical vertebroplasty

Vertebroplasty in the cervical spine is uncommon but can be performed with a 15-gauge needle via transpedicular or anterolateral approaches. Vertebroplasty of odontoid fractures has been performed successfully with

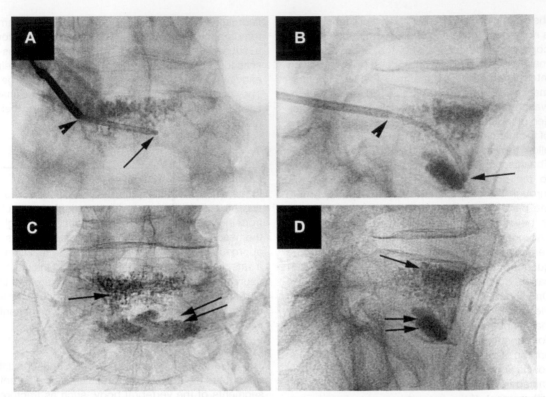

Fig. 7. Curved needle vertebroplasty allowing targeting of an unfilled fracture cleft. The guiding needle tip (*arrow*) is in the left posterolateral vertebral body (*arrowhead*), and the curved nitinol needle is directed to the (*A*) mid and (*B*) inferior zones of the vertebra. (*C, D*) Trabecular cement filling pattern in the superior body (*arrow*) and separate homogenous cement filling of an inferior fracture cleft (*double arrow*). (*Images courtesy of* Dr. Albert J. Yoo, Division of Interventional Neuroradiology, Massachusetts General Hospital, Boston, MA).

a transoral approach under general anesthesia by both regular fluoroscopic[46] and CT-guided methods.[47] Antiseptic preparation of the oropharynx, a coaxial system, and intravenous antibiotics seem to give satisfactory coverage against contamination by oral flora.

Pathologic fractures

Vertebroplasty can be used to treat pathologic fractures including those caused by inoperable malignant (myeloma, metastases) or benign (eg, hemangioma) lesions.[48] If the diagnosis is uncertain, it is important first to take biopsies of the lesion for assessment. Treating these lesions has an increased risk because of the greater propensity for a soft tissue lesion to be displaced by the cement infusion, particularly if the lesion involves the posterior wall of the body (**Fig. 8**). If the lesion already extends into the spinal canal, extreme care is required, and it may be better to avoid vertebroplasty altogether. Complications related to cement extravasation occur in up to 10% of these cases.[49] Some operators perform a tumor ablation via a radiofrequency probe advanced through the

vertebroplasty needle, followed by vertebroplasty.[28,29,50] The heat generated during ablation can cause neural damage if the tumor is adjacent to nerve roots or the cord. More refined bipolar radiofrequency probes use circulating saline to maintain a tighter core of thermoablation.[51] Laser-induced thermotherapy[52] and plasma ablation[53] are more recent modalities that create a targeted cavity in the tumor.

Lordoplasty

Described by Heini and Orler[54] in 2004 and by Orler and colleagues[55] in 2006, lordoplasty has been proposed as a cost-effective method of achieving height restoration. In addition to the compressed vertebra, bipedicular access is performed in the levels immediately above and below. These two vertebrae are reinforced with cement; then the trocars are reinserted into the needles, and the handles are brought together from above and below to reduce kyphotic angulation and to distract the fractured vertebra. Cement then is injected into the fracture while it is distracted. The authors report an average correction in angulation

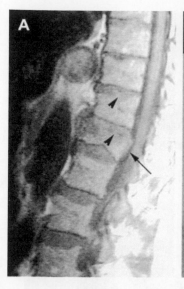
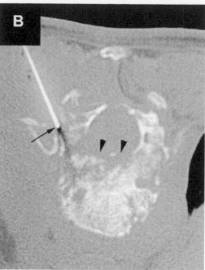

Fig. 8. (*A*) Pathologic fractures with destruction of the endplates of adjacent vertebrae (*arrowheads*) and extension into the anterior canal on T1 MRI (*arrow*). (*B*) The needle (*arrow*) was guided by CT because the pedicle was poorly visualized under fluoroscopy. Note posterior cortical destruction (*arrowheads*). The patient was transferred to the fluoroscopy suite for the cement injection.

of 14° in 30 cases. The procedure is painful and requires general anesthesia.

Sacroplasty

Sacroplasty provides palliation and speeds mobilization after insufficiency and traumatic fractures of the sacral alae. It can be performed using the dual-modality approach of CT-guided needle placement followed by transfer to the fluoroscopy unit for cement injection (**Fig. 9**). Usually two needles, one superior and one inferior, are advanced perpendicularly down onto the fracture line. If the fractures are bilateral, both sides can be treated in the same session. Because of the orientation of the sacral ala, the hubs of the contralateral needles angle medially and can impinge on each other. Using needles with smaller handles at the hub helps limit this imposition. An alternative technique is performed entirely under fluoroscopy and involves guiding the needles along the line of the fracture from inferior to superior, staying lateral to the sacral foraminae and medial to the sacroiliac joints (**Fig. 10**). This technique is technically more challenging because of the complex landmarks provided by the curved sacroiliac joints and sacral foraminae.

Kyphoplasty

Kyphoplasty (Medtronic, Minneapolis, Minnesota) is a modification approved by the Food and Drug Administration in 1998, involving the use of an inflatable balloon to create a cavity in the bone and reduce the pressure of the cement injection.[56] Although initially reported to offer possible height restoration,[57] this effect usually is subtle, at best, in general use. Kyphoplasty has been shown to

have a lower rate of cement leakage,[58,59] making it advantageous in cases with tumor infiltration and a compromised posterior vertebral margin. Detrimental tumor displacement still can occur during the balloon inflations, however. The pattern of balloon expansion can be unpredictable, and the balloon occasionally can herniate through the endplate. Overall, the efficacy of kyphoplasty in providing pain relief is similar to that of vertebroplasty.[59] The main disadvantages are its relatively high cost, the use of a larger needle (previously 8 gauge but now available as a 10-gauge system), the need for bipedicular access, and the typical requirement for general anesthesia.

Skyphoplasty

The Sky Bone Expander polymer device (Disc-O-Tech, Monroe, New Jersey) creates a vertebral cavity in a similar fashion to the kyphoplasty device. Instead of using balloon inflation, the device employs a plastic tube with longitudinal slits that has a low profile along a delivery rod when elongated but forms a tightly calibrated (14 or 16 mm) mulberry-shaped ball created by a concertina/accordion effect when it is pushed through the cannula.[60] The mechanism is reversed to wind the tube back into a low, elongated profile before removing the probe. The device has an outer profile of 4 mm. There are limited descriptions of its use, although it seems to provide results similar to those obtained with the Kyphon system.[21]

Complications and Pitfalls

Reported complications rates are in the range of 1% to 2% for osteoporotic fractures and 5% to 10% for neoplastic fractures.[61–71]

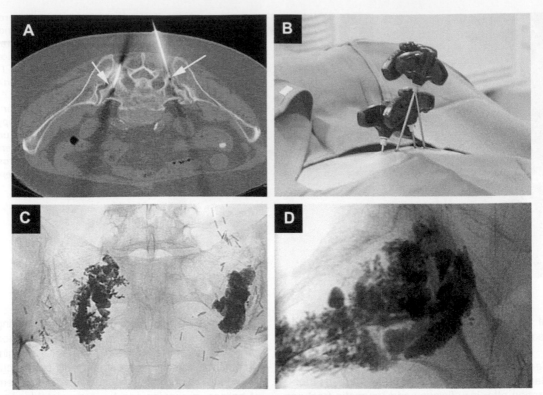

Fig. 9. (*A*) Sacroplasty with CT-guided needle placement (*arrows*). (*B*) Needles in situ after CT placement and transfer to the fluoroscopy suite. Note how the handles angle toward each other. (*C*) Anteroposterior and (*D*) lateral views of cement distributed through both sacral alae.

Needle injury

Aberrant needle passage must be avoided by recognizing the critical fluoroscopic landmarks described earlier in this article. Direct injuries can occur to the exiting nerve root, to the thecal sac with cerebrospinal fluid leak, to the spinal cord, to the pleural space with pneumothorax, or to the aorta with severe hemorrhage (see **Fig. 4**). It is possible to cause new fractures of the posterior elements with aggressive torquing of the needle.

Cement migration

Cement can migrate through fissures in the wall of the vertebral body, through the endplates into the disc space (**Fig. 11**), anteriorly into the prevertebral space (**Fig. 12**), posterolaterally into the intervertebral foramen, or posteriorly into the epidural space (**Figs. 12** and **13**). Significant (symptomatic) leaks into the spinal canal are rare, with none reported in one series of more than 1000 patients;[72] however, the consequences can be devastating with intractable pain and neurologic deficits.[73] Most of the benefit and increased stability afforded by vertebroplasty is accrued from filling the anterior portion of the

vertebral body, which is the part most liable to undergo further compression. There is little extra advantage to be gained by attempting aggressively to fill more of the vertebra and allowing cement to migrate into the posterior quarter of the body (**Fig. 14**). Cement migration into the disc space is avoided because it alters the spinal biomechanics unfavorably, placing the adjacent vertebrae at greater risk of fracture.[74] This migration, however, occurs in up to 10% of cases, and small volumes are tolerated well.[75] Fenestration of the pedicular cortex or use of the parapedicular approach increases the risk of cement leaking out along the needle track. Published reports of cement leaks are variable, given the reliance of many reports on the use of plain radiographs for postprocedural assessment.[59] Radiographs have been shown to have a sensitivity of only 48% compared with the nearly 100% sensitivity of a postprocedure CT.[76] In fact, postprocedure CT assessment reveals tiny asymptomatic foci of cement in paravertebral veins in the majority of cases. The rate of symptomatic migration is more relevant and should be less than 1% to 2%.[59]

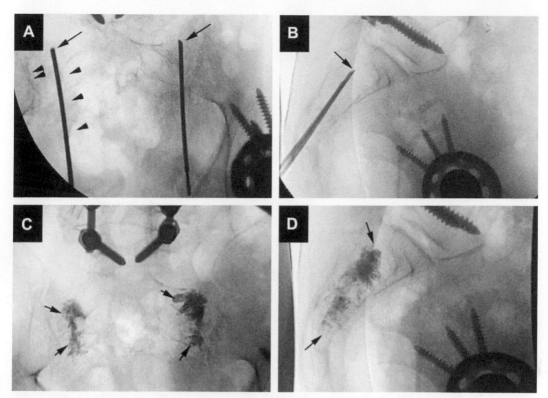

Fig. 10. Sacroplasty with fluoroscopic control throughout. Bilateral needle placement (*A*) parallel to and (*B*) between the sacral foraminae (*arrowheads*) and SI joints (*double arrowhead*) with distal tips (*arrows*). Optimal cement distribution in the sacral ala adjacent to the SI joints (*arrows*) on (*C*) AP and (*D*) lateral projections. (*Images courtesy of* Dr. Manraj K.S. Heran, Department of Radiology, Vancouver General Hospital, Vancouver, British Columbia, Canada.)

Pulmonary embolism

Emboli can be caused by cement, marrow, or air entering the vertebral venous system via the basivertebral and paravertebral veins (**Fig. 15**).[77–80] During the cement injection, marrow embolism is invisible on fluoroscopy, air is unlikely to be detected, and even cement can go unnoticed if

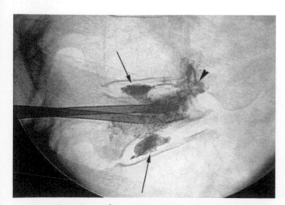

Fig. 11. Migration of cement into both adjacent discs (*arrows*) and into the prevertebral space (*arrowhead*).

washed out rapidly by blood flow. In large series of 532 patients, there was a 2.1% incidence of radiographic cement embolism; none of the instances were symptomatic.[81] Fatal pulmonary emboli have been reported, and the risk of significant adverse events increases with multilevel treatments, probably because of a cumulative effect of multiple marrow microemboli. Vertebral corporeal venography (**Fig. 6**), performed through the vertebroplasty needle, was in vogue in the early years of the procedure, but operators found the results did not predict emboli or significantly alter the conduct of the procedure.

Infection

Pyogenic spondylitis after vertebroplasty is rare, with only a small number of case reports published.[49,82] Symptoms are nonspecific relapse of severe back pain and tend to present about a year after treatment. Patients should be worked up with laboratory sedimentation rate and C-reactive protein level, as well as undergoing a contrast-enhanced MRI scan. Treatment often requires

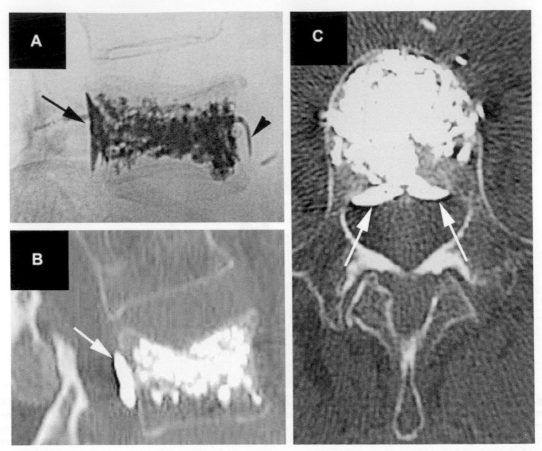

Fig. 12. Cement migration into the epidural space (*arrows*) on (*A*) fluoroscopy and (*B, C*) CT. Arrowhead in *A* indicates prevertebral venous penetration.

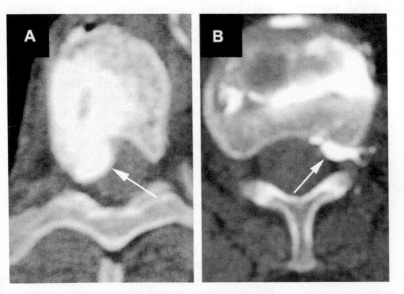

Fig. 13. CT demonstration of (*A*) right paracentral cement migration indenting the thecal sac (*arrow*) and (*B*) left epidural and foraminal migration compromising the left exiting nerve root (*arrow*).

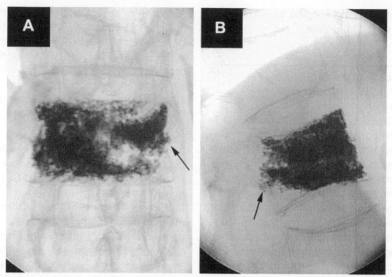

Fig. 14. Aggressive filling of this vertebra to (*A*) the bilateral margins (*arrow*) and (*B*) posterior surface (*arrow*) should be avoided because of the dubious additional benefit and increased risk.

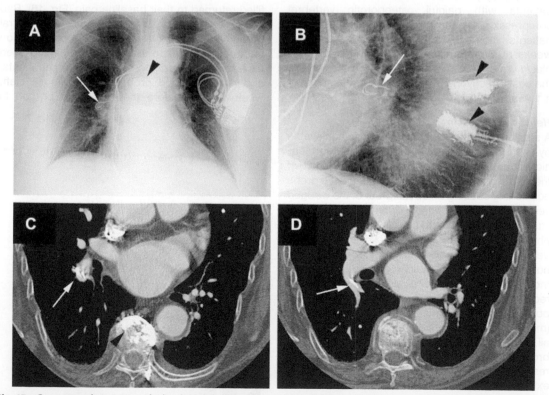

Fig. 15. Cement pulmonary embolus (*arrow*) demonstrated in the right interlobar pulmonary artery on (*A*) anteroposterior and (*B*) lateral chest radiographs and on (*C, D*) dynamic intravenous contrast-enhanced CT. Note vertebroplasty of two thoracic vertebral bodies (*arrowheads* in *A* and *B*).

surgical debridement and fixation in addition to intravenous antibiotic treatment.

Controversies

Long-term efficacy of percutaneous vertebroplasty versus conventional medical therapy

After 20 years there is still, at best, only level III evidence consisting of nonrandomized comparisons between vertebroplasty and medical therapy to support an added benefit of vertebroplasty. A randomized, controlled trial is in progress, however. The Investigational Vertebroplasty Efficacy and Safety Trial (INVEST)[83] hopes to recruit 166 patients over 5 years from multiple centers. Patients will be assigned randomly to undergo either vertebroplasty or a control intervention. The control consists of a sham procedure including the same sterile preparation, local anesthetic infiltration down to the pedicle, and skin incision, but thereafter the operator merely palpates the skin to simulate manipulation of a vertebroplasty needle. Both patients and patient evaluators are blinded as to the type of intervention. Primary outcome will be pain relief at 1 month.

Another randomized study of "percutaneous vertebroplasty versus conservative therapy in patients with painful osteoporotic vertebral compression fractures," VERTOS II, will assign patients who have insufficiency fractures within 6 weeks of symptom onset randomly to vertebroplasty or conservative treatment and will compare the cost effectiveness of the two approaches over a 1-year period.[84]

Height restoration

A small degree of height restoration is achievable by both vertebroplasty and the augmented techniques described in previous sections. Much of the height gain is generated by the patient's prone positioning causing an opening-out of the wedged vertebrae before cement fixation.[85] Cadaveric studies have shown additional height gain with kyphoplasty ex vivo.[86,87] Several clinical series also demonstrated improved height with kyphoplasty but relied on lateral radiographs rather than on more definitive CT or MR assessment.[85,88,89] A recent study comparing preprocedure MR with postprocedure CT studies demonstrated a small (mean, 1–2 mm) increase in vertebral height overall, with no significant difference between vertebroplasty and kyphoplasty.[90] Although height restoration has not been shown to provide any extra improvement in pain relief,[91] it may be valuable in certain circumstances, such as kyphosis that causes restrictive pulmonary failure.[92] Special efforts can be made when positioning the patient

to maximize reduction of the deformity or by modifying the kyphoplasty technique by keeping one balloon inflated while filling the contralateral cavity with cement. Lordoplasty, described earlier, is relatively invasive and has limited reports, although an average anterior height increase of 10 mm was described in a series of 26 patients.[55]

Filling the cleft

Fracture clefts, thought to be related to avascular necrosis or fracture non-union with vacuum phenomenon, were described first on plain radiographs as linear gas-filled lesions usually adjacent to an endplate and with detectable motion at the cleft on fluoroscopy.[93] Linear T2 hyperintensities seen on MR are considered to be fluid-filled versions of the same lesion. Although a pattern of cement filling a cleft is visualized during approximately one third of vertebroplasties, only half of these are detected prospectively on preprocedure MR,[94] possibly because clefts become more obvious when the spine is extended in the prone position. Lane and colleagues[94] found a nonstatistically significant trend toward better pain relief in patients who had a cleft filled during vertebroplasty compared with those who had no cleft, and all four patients who had a cleft that was not filled returned to their baseline pain (**Fig. 16**). Rad and colleagues[95] recommend targeting the central portion of severe (vertebra plana) compression fractures, counter to the accepted method used for less severely compressed lateral components, and report a good probability of filling a cleft, whether seen before the procedure or not. In

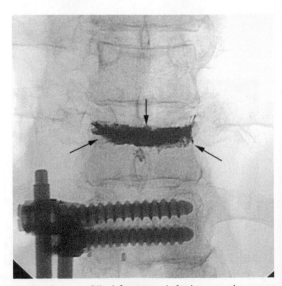

Fig. 16. Cement-filled fracture cleft deep to the superior endplate (*arrows*).

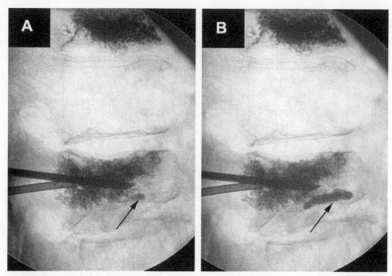

Fig. 17. (*A, B*) Penetration of inferior fracture cleft (*arrow*) without need to reposition needle.

general, however, it is not necessary to target the cleft directly, because the cement usually enters the cleft freely via adjacent fissures (**Fig. 17**). If the cleft remains unfilled, an attempt can be made to reposition the needle, or a second needle can be advanced into the cleft through the contralateral pedicle. Altered biomechanics from cement-filled clefts may create a higher risk of a subsequent adjacent vertebral fracture than associated with a vertebroplasty without cleft filling.[96]

Potential increased risk of adjacent compression fractures

Vertebroplasty hardens and reduces the compliance of the vertebral body, alters the biomechanical balance within the spinal column, and transfers forces directly to the adjacent level.[63,97] Intuitively one would expect the adjacent vertebrae to be at increased risk of subsequent collapse, and this expectation seems to be borne out by a number of observational studies[98,99] showing the rate of fractures at these levels to be increased up to threefold. A causal relationship is supported further by the large proportion of otherwise rare inferior endplate fractures in the vertebra immediately above the treated level. As reported by Trout and Kallmes,[100] however, the overall rate of subsequent vertebral fracture is comparable to the 19.2% rate expected in the osteoporotic spine regardless of vertebroplasty.[21] The tendency for adjacent levels to be affected may reflect the typical clustering of insufficiency fractures around the thoracolumbar region. It is hoped that a randomized trial can help to answer this question.

Vertebroplasty versus kyphoplasty

The debate regarding the relative merits of vertebroplasty and kyphoplasty continues. Proponents of kyphoplasty point to a more controlled procedure with lower rates of cement migration and a questionably greater potential for height restoration. Vertebroplasty, however, is a faster, more straightforward, less invasive, and cheaper procedure that has not been shown to give inferior results,[101] and the increased rate of cement migration does not result in increased morbidity. After almost 20 years, the lack of a randomized comparison between the main alternatives in vertebral augmentation ensures that the debate will continue.

SUMMARY

Vertebroplasty now is an established part of the treatment algorithm for vertebral fractures because of its consistent effectiveness in ameliorating debilitating pain and breaking the cycle of pain and deconditioning. It is a safe procedure when performed meticulously with a sound understanding of the relevant anatomy, technique, and goals. The lack of level I evidence for its benefit may be addressed by a randomized, blinded, controlled trial in the near future.

ACKNOWLEDGMENTS

The authors express their appreciation to Dr. Manraj K.S. Heran, Dr. Albert J. Woo, and Dr. Benjamin Liu for their valued contributions to this article.

REFERENCES

1. Galibert P, Deramond H, Rosat P, et al. Preliminary note on the treatment of vertebral angioma by percutaneous acrylic vertebroplasty. Neurochirurgie 1987;33(2):166–8.

2. Ray NF, Chan JK, Thamer M, et al. Medical expenditures for the treatment of osteoporotic fractures in the United States in 1995: report from the National Osteoporosis Foundation. J Bone Miner Res 1997; 12(1):24–35.

3. Melton LJ. Epidemiology of spinal osteoporosis. Spine 1997;22(Suppl 24):2S–11S.

4. Old JL, Calvert M. Vertebral compression fractures in the elderly. Am Fam Physician 2004;69: 111–6.

5. Riggs BL, Melton LJ III. The worldwide problem of osteoporosis: insights afforded by epidemiology. Bone 1995;17(5 Suppl):505–11.

6. NIH Consensus Development Panel on Osteoporosis Prevention, Diagnosis, and Therapy. Osteoporosis prevention, diagnosis, and therapy. JAMA 2001;285:785–95, 2008.

7. van Staa TP, Leufkens HGM, Abenhaim L, et al. Use of oral corticosteroids and risk of fractures. J Bone Miner Res 2000;15:993–1000.

8. Lau E, Ong K, Kurtz S, et al. Mortality following the diagnosis of a vertebral compression fracture in the Medicare population. J Bone Joint Surg Am 2008; 90(7):1479–86.

9. Jackson SA, Tenenhouse A, Robertson L. Vertebral fractures definition from population-based data: preliminary results from the Canadian Multicenter Osteoporosis Study (CaMos). Osteoporos Int 2000;11:680–7.

10. Papaioannou A, Watts NB, Kendler DL. Diagnosis and management of vertebral fractures in elderly adults. Am J Med 2002;113:220–8.

11. Cooper C, Atkinson EJ, Jacobson SJ, et al. Population-based study of survival after osteoporotic fractures. Am J Epidemiol 1993;137:1001–5.

12. Schlaich C, Minne HW, Bruckner T, et al. Reduced pulmonary function in patients with spinal osteoporotic fractures. Osteoporos Int 1998;8:261–7.

13. Lukert BP. Vertebral compression fractures: how to manage pain, avoid disability. Geriatrics 1994;49: 22–6.

14. Lyles KW. Management of patients with vertebral compression fractures. Pharmacotherapy 1999; 19(1 Pt 2):21s–4s.

15. Wu SS, Lachmann E, Nagler W. Current medical, rehabilitation, and surgical management of vertebral compression fractures. J Womens Health (Larchmt) 2003;12(1):17–26.

16. Tezer M, Erturer RE, Ozturk C, et al. Conservative treatment of fractures of the thoracolumbar spine. Int Orthop 2005;29:78–82.

17. Silverman SL. The clinical consequences of vertebral compression fracture. Bone 2009;13(Suppl 2):27–31.

18. Gold DT. The clinical impact of vertebral fractures: quality of life in women with osteoporosis. Bone 1996;18(Suppl 3):185–9.

19. Convertino VA, Bloomfield SA, Greenleaf JF. An overview of the issues: physiological effects of bed rest and restricted physical activity. Med Sci Sports Exerc 1997;29:187–90.

20. Lieberman I, Reinhardt MK. Vertebroplasty and kyphoplasty for osteolytic vertebral collapse. Clin Orthop Relat Res 2003;415:176–86.

21. Lindsay R, Silverman SL, Cooper C, et al. Risk of new vertebral fracture in the year following a fracture. JAMA 2001;285(3):320–3.

22. Kearns AE, Kallmes DF. Osteoporosis primer for the vertebroplasty practitioner: expanding the focus beyond needles and cement. AJNR Am J Neuroradiol 2008;29:1816–22.

23. Friedrich M, Gittler G, Pieler-Bruha E. Misleading history of pain location in 51 patients with osteoporotic vertebral fractures. Eur Spine J 2006;15(12): 1797–800.

24. Gaughen JR Jr, Jensen ME, Schweickert PA, et al. Lack of preoperative spinous process tenderness does not affect clinical success of percutaneous vertebroplasty. J Vasc Interv Radiol 2002;13: 1135–8.

25. Li JM. Pain management in the hospitalized patient. Med Clin North Am 2002;86(4):771–95.

26. Cotten A, Dewatre F, Cortet B, et al. Percutaneous vertebroplasty for osteolytic metastases and myeloma: effects of the percentage of lesion filling and the leakage of methyl methacrylate at clinical follow-up. Radiology 1996;200:525–30.

27. Weill A, Chiras J, Simon JM, et al. Spinal metastases: indications for and results of percutaneous injection of acrylic surgical cement. Radiology 1996;199(1):241–7.

28. Halpin RJ, Bendok BR, Liu JC. Minimally invasive treatments for spinal metastases: vertebroplasty, kyphoplasty, and radiofrequency ablation. J Support Oncol 2004;2:339–51.

29. van der LE, Kroft LJ, Dijkstra PD. Treatment of vertebral tumor with posterior wall defect using image-guided radiofrequency ablation combined with vertebroplasty: preliminary results in 12 patients. J Vasc Interv Radiol 2007;18:741–7.

30. Campbell SE, Phillips CD, Dubovsky E, et al. The value of CT in determining potential instability of simple wedge-compression fractures of the lumbar spine. AJNR Am J Neuroradiol 1995;16(7):1385–92.

31. Tanigawa N, Komemushi A, Kariya S, et al. Percutaneous vertebroplasty: relationship between vertebral body bone marrow edema pattern on MR images and initial clinical response. Radiology 2006;239:195–200.

32. Yang X, Mi S, Mahadevia AA, et al. Pain reduction in osteoporotic patients with vertebral pain without measurable compression. Neuroradiology 2008; 50(2):153–9.

33. Uemura A, Kobayashi N, Numaguchi Y, et al. Preprocedural MR imaging for percutaneous vertebroplasty: special interest in contrast enhancement. Radiat Med 2007;25:325–8.

34. Hsu CY, Yu CW, Wu MZ, et al. Unusual manifestations of vertebral osteomyelitis: intraosseous lesions mimicking metastases. AJNR Am J Neuroradiol 2008;29(6):1104–10.

35. Hiwatashi A, Ohigiya Y, Kakimoto N, et al. Cement leakage during vertebroplasty can be predicted on preoperative MRI. AJR Am J Roentgenol 2007; 188(4):1089–93.

36. Maynard AS, Jensen ME, Schweickert PA, et al. Value of bone scan imaging in predicting pain relief from percutaneous vertebroplasty in osteoporotic vertebral fractures. AJNR Am J Neuroradiol 2000; 21:1807–12.

37. Masala S, Schillaci O, Massari F, et al. MRI and bone scan imaging in the preoperative evaluation of painful vertebral fractures treated with vertebroplasty and kyphoplasty. In Vivo 2005;19:1055–60.

38. Luginbuhl M. Percutaneous vertebroplasty, kyphoplasty and lordoplasty: implications for the anesthesiologist. Curr Opin Anaesthesiol 2008;21: 504–13.

39. Ekstein M, Gavish D, Ezri T, et al. Monitored anaesthesia care in the elderly: guidelines and recommendations. Drugs Aging 2008;25(6): 477–500.

40. Hiwatashi A, Yoshiura T, Noguchi T, et al. Usefulness of cone-beam CT before and after percutaneous vertebroplasty. AJR Am J Roentgenol 2008;191:1401–5.

41. Murphy KJ, Lin DD, Khan AA, et al. Multilevel vertebroplasty via a single pedicular approach using a curved 13-gauge needle: technical note. Can Assoc Radiol J 2002;53:293–5.

42. Brook AL, Miller TS, Fast A, et al. Vertebral augmentation with a flexible curved needle: preliminary results in 17 consecutive patients. J Vasc Interv Radiol 2009;19(12):1785–9.

43. Kwon YJ. Modified vertebroplasty using a curved probe: technique and preliminary results. Minim Invasive Neurosurg 2008;51:187–91.

44. Kim JH, Park KS, Yi S, et al. Real-time CT fluoroscopy (CTF)-guided vertebroplasty in osteoporotic spine fractures. Yonsei Med J 2005;46: 635–42.

45. Trumm CG, Jakobs TF, Zech CJ, et al. CT fluoroscopy-guided percutaneous vertebroplasty for the treatment of osteolytic breast cancer metastases: results in 62 sessions with 86 vertebrae treated. J Vasc Interv Radiol 2008;19:1596–606.

46. Gailloud P, Martin JB, Olivi A, et al. Transoral vertebroplasty for a fractured C2 aneurysmal bone cyst. J Vasc Interv Radiol 2002;13:340–1.

47. Reddy AS, Hochman M, Loh S, et al. CT guided direct transoral approach to C2 for percutaneous vertebroplasty. Pain Physician 2005;8:235–8.

48. Georgy BA. Metastatic spinal lesions: state-of-the-art treatment options and future trends. AJNR Am J Neuroradiol 2008;29(9):1605–11.

49. Chiras J, Depriester C, Weill A, et al. Percutaneous vertebral surgery: techniques and indications. J Neuroradiol 1997;24:45–59 [in French].

50. Gronemeyer DH, Schirp S, Gevargez A. Image-guided radiofrequency ablation of spinal tumors: preliminary experience with an expandable array electrode. Cancer J 2002;8:33–9.

51. Buy X, Basile A, Bierry G, et al. Saline-infused bipolar radiofrequency ablation of high-risk spinal and paraspinal neoplasms. AJR Am J Roentgenol 2006;186(5 Suppl):S322–6.

52. Ahn H, Mousavi P, Chin L, et al. The effect of pre-vertebroplasty tumor ablation using laser-induced thermotherapy on biomechanical stability and cement fill in the metastatic spine. Eur Spine J 2007;16(8):1171–8.

53. Georgy BA, Wong W. Plasma-mediated radiofrequency ablation assisted percutaneous cement injection for treating advanced malignant vertebral compression fractures. AJNR Am J Neuroradiol 2007;28:700–5.

54. Heini PF, Orler R. Kyphoplasty for treatment of osteoporotic vertebral fractures. Eur Spine J 2004; 13(3):184–92.

55. Orler R, Frauchiger LH, Lange U, et al. Lordoplasty: report on early results with a new technique for the treatment of vertebral compression fractures to restore the lordosis. Eur Spine J 2006;15(12): 1769–75.

56. Weisskopf M, Ohnsorge JA, Niethard FU. Intravertebral pressure during vertebroplasty and balloon kyphoplasty: an in vitro study. Spine 2008;33:178–82.

57. Garfin SR, Yuan HA, Reiley MA. Kyphoplasty and vertebroplasty for the treatment of painful osteoporotic compression fractures. Spine 2001;26(14):1511–5.

58. Taylor RS, Taylor RJ, Fritzell P. Balloon kyphoplasty and vertebroplasty for vertebral compression fractures: a comparative systematic review of efficacy and safety. Spine 2006;31:2747–55.

59. Eck JC, Nachtigall D, Humphreys SC, et al. Comparison of vertebroplasty and balloon kyphoplasty for treatment of vertebral compression fractures: a meta-analysis of the literature. Spine J 2008;8:488–97.

60. Peh WC, Munk PL, Rashid F, et al. Percutaneous vertebral augmentation: vertebroplasty, kyphoplasty and kkyphoplasty. Radiol Clin North Am 2008;46:611–35, vii.

61. McGraw JK, Cardella J, Barr JD, et al. Society of Interventional Radiology quality improvement guidelines for percutaneous vertebroplasty. J Vasc Interv Radiol 2003;14:S311–5.

62. Padovani B, Kasriel O, Brunner P, et al. Pulmonary embolism caused by acrylic cement: a rare complication of percutaneous vertebroplasty. AJNR Am J Neuroradiol 1999;20:375–7.

63. Jensen ME, Evans AJ, Mathis JM, et al. Percutaneous polymethylmethacrylate vertebroplasty in the treatment of osteoporotic vertebral body compression fracture: technical aspects. AJNR Am J Neuroradiol 1997;18:1897–904.

64. Choe du H, Marom EM, Ahrar K, et al. Pulmonary embolism of polymethyl methacrylate during percutaneous vertebroplasty and kyphoplasty. AJR Am J Roentgenol 2004;183:1097–102.

65. Ratliff J, Nguyen J, Heiss J. Root and spinal cord compression from methylmethacrylate vertebroplasty. Spine 2001;26:E300–2.

66. Deramond H, Depriester C, Galibert P, et al. Percutaneous vertebroplasty with polymethylmethacrylate. Radiol Clin North Am 1998;36:533–46.

67. Barr JD, Barr MS, Lemley TJ, et al. Percutaneous vertebroplasty for pain relief and spinal stabilization. Spine 2000;25:923–8.

68. Harrington KD. Major neurological complications following percutaneous vertebroplasty with polymethylmethacrylate: a case report. J Bone Joint Surg Am 2001;83-A:1070–3.

69. Lee BJ, Lee SR, Yoo TY. Paraplegia as a complication of percutaneous vertebroplasty with polymethylmethacrylate: a case report. Spine 2002;27:E419–22.

70. Jang JS, Lee SH, Jung SK. Pulmonary embolism of polymethylmethacrylate after percutaneous vertebroplasty: a report of three cases. Spine 2002;27:E416–8.

71. Vasconcelos C, Gailloud P, Martin JB, et al. Transient arterial hypotension induced by polymethylmethacrylate injection during percutaneous vertebroplasty. J Vasc Interv Radiol 2001;12:1001–2.

72. Masala S, Mastrangeli R, Petrella MC, et al. Percutaneous vertebroplasty in 1,253 levels: results and long-term effectiveness in a single centre. Eur Radiol 2009;19(1):165–71.

73. Teng MM, Cheng H, Ho DM, et al. Intraspinal leakage of bone cement after vertebroplasty: a report of 3 cases. AJNR Am J Neuroradiol 2006;27(1):224–9.

74. Lin EP, Ekholm S, Hiwatashi A, et al. Vertebroplasty: cement leakage into the disc increases the risk of new fracture of adjacent vertebral body. AJNR Am J Neuroradiol 2004;25:175–80.

75. Syed MI, Patel NA, Jan S, et al. Intradiskal extravasation with low-volume cement filling in percutaneous vertebroplasty. AJNR Am J Neuroradiol 2005;26:2397–401.

76. Schmidt R, Cakir B, Mattes T, et al. Cement leakage during vertebroplasty: an underestimated problem? Eur Spine J 2005;14:466–73.

77. Ramos L, de Las Heras JA, Sanchez S, et al. Medium-term results of percutaneous vertebroplasty in multiple myeloma. Eur J Haematol 2006; 77:7–13.

78. Barragan-Campos HM, Vallee JN, Lo D, et al. Percutaneous vertebroplasty for spinal metastases: complications. Radiology 2006;238:354–62.

79. Krauss M, Hirschfelder H, Tomandl B, et al. Kyphosis reduction and the rate of cement leaks after vertebroplasty of intravertebral clefts. Eur Radiol 2006;16:1015–21.

80. Mousavi P, Roth S, Finkelstein J, et al. Volumetric quantification of cement leakage following percutaneous vertebroplasty in metastatic and osteoporotic vertebrae. J Neurosurg 2003;99:56–9.

81. Venmans A, Lohle PN, van Rooij WJ, et al. Frequency and outcome of pulmonary polymethylmethacrylate embolism during percutaneous vertebroplasty. AJNR Am J Neuroradiol 2008;29:1983–5.

82. Shin JH, Ha KY, Kim KW, et al. Surgical treatment for delayed pyogenic spondylitis after percutaneous vertebroplasty and kyphoplasty. Report of 4 cases. J Neurosurg Spine 2008;9:265–72.

83. Gray LA, Jarvik JG, Heagerty PJ, et al. INvestigational Vertebroplasty Efficacy and Safety Trial (INVEST): a randomized controlled trial of percutaneous vertebroplasty. BMC Musculoskelet Disord 2007;8:126.

84. Klazen C, Verhaar H, Lampmann L, et al. VERTOS II: percutaneous vertebroplasty versus conservative therapy in patients with painful osteoporotic vertebral compression fractures; rationale, objectives and design of a multicenter randomized controlled trial. Trials 2007;8(1):33.

85. Voggenreiter G. Balloon kyphoplasty is effective in deformity correction of osteoporotic vertebral compression fractures. Spine 2009;30(24):2806–12.

86. Hiwatashi A, Sidhu R, Lee RK, et al. Kyphoplasty versus vertebroplasty to increase vertebral body height: a cadaveric study. Radiology 2005;237: 1115–9.

87. Belkoff SM, Mathis JM, Fenton DC, et al. An ex vivo biomechanical evaluation of an inflatable bone tamp used in the treatment of compression fracture. Spine 2001;26(2):151–6.

88. Ledlie JT, Renfro M. Balloon kyphoplasty: one-year outcomes in vertebral body height restoration, chronic pain, and activity levels. J Neurosurg 2003;98:S36–42.

89. Rhyne A, Banit D, Laxer E, et al. Kyphoplasty: report of eighty-two thoracolumbar osteoporotic vertebral fractures. J Orthop Trauma 2004;18(5):294–9.

90. Hiwatashi A, Westesson PL, Yoshiura T, et al. Kyphoplasty and vertebroplasty produce the

same degree of height restoration. AJNR Am J Neuroradiol 2009; in press.

91. McKiernan F, Faciszewski T, Jensen R. Does vertebral height restoration achieved at vertebroplasty matter? J Vasc Interv Radiol 2005;16:973–9.

92. Tanigawa N, Kariya S, Kojima H, et al. Improvement in respiratory function by percutaneous vertebroplasty. Acta Radiol 2008;49:638–43.

93. Maladague BE, Noel HM, Malghem JJ. The intravertebral vacuum cleft: a sign of ischemic vertebral collapse. Radiology 1978;129(1):23–9.

94. Lane JI, Maus TP, Wald JT, et al. Intravertebral clefts opacified during vertebroplasty: pathogenesis, technical implications, and prognostic significance. AJNR Am J Neuroradiol 2002;23(10):1642–6.

95. Rad AE, Gray LA, Kallmes DF. Significance and targeting of small, central clefts in severe fractures treated with vertebroplasty. AJNR Am J Neuroradiol 2008;29(7):1285–7.

96. Trout AT, Kallmes DF, Lane JI, et al. Subsequent vertebral fractures after vertebroplasty: association with intraosseous clefts. AJNR Am J Neuroradiol 2006;27:1586–91.

97. Berlemann U, Ferguson SJ, Nolte LP, et al. Adjacent vertebral failure after vertebroplasty. A biomechanical investigation. J Bone Joint Surg Br 2002;84:748–52.

98. Grados F, Depriester C, Cayrolle G, et al. Long-term observations of vertebral osteoporotic fractures treated by percutaneous vertebroplasty. Rheumatology (Oxford) 2000;39:1410–4.

99. Kim SH, Kang HS, Choi JA, et al. Risk factors of new compression fractures in adjacent vertebrae after percutaneous vertebroplasty. Acta Radiol 2004;45:440–5.

100. Trout AT, Kallmes DF. Does vertebroplasty cause incident vertebral fractures? A review of available data. AJNR Am J Neuroradiol 2006;27:1397–403.

101. Pflugmacher R, Kandziora F, Schroder R, et al. [Vertebroplasty and kyphoplasty in osteoporotic fractures of vertebral bodies—a prospective 1-year follow-up analysis]. Rofo 2005;177:1670–6 [in German].

Inferior Petrosal Sinus Sampling in the Diagnosis of Sellar Neuropathology

Nestor D. Tomycz, MD[a,b], Michael B. Horowitz, MD[a,b],*

KEYWORDS
- Cushing's disease • Hypercortisolism • Pituitary
- Cushing's syndrome • Sella • Endovascular

Cushing's disease (CD) is hypercortisolism engendered by a corticotropin (ACTH)-secreting pituitary tumor. The phenotype of cortisol excess is shared by numerous other hyperplastic/tumorigenic disorders that are included in the blanket term "Cushing's syndrome" (CS). Moreover, iatrogenic cortisol excess from glucocorticoid administration and pseudo-Cushing states associated with alcoholism and depression can mimic the clinical and biochemical characteristics of CS. Once CS and ACTH dependence have been established, further tests are mandatory to determine whether the neoplastic cause of excess ACTH secretion is pituitary (CD) or ectopic. Because no single test is definitive for CD, establishing the diagnosis has remained a challenge that relies on building a critical mass of evidence. The differential diagnosis of ACTH-dependent CS traditionally has rested on noninvasive biochemical and radiologic testing. Bilateral inferior petrosal sinus sampling (BIPSS) is an invasive procedure that has become part of the diagnostic armamentarium surrounding CD. When used appropriately—that is, for patients who have biochemically confirmed ACTH-dependent CS but discordant biochemical or radiologic studies—BIPSS is the reference standard confirmatory test for CD.

CLINICAL BACKGROUND

Supraphysiologic exposure to cortisol causes a distinct constellation of symptoms and signs: decreased libido, weight gain, moon facies, hypertension, glucose intolerance or diabetes mellitus type 2, plethoric facies, reddish striae, hirsutism, menstrual dysfunction, muscle weakness, easy bruising, thinning of the skin, growth retardation in children, and neuropsychologic disturbances such as depression.[1] The primary screening tests for hypercortisolism include the 24-hour urinary free cortisol, late-night salivary cortisol, and the low-dose dexamethasone suppression tests. Once hypercortisolism (ie, CS) is established and pseudo-Cushing's states are ruled out, checking a plasma ACTH helps subclassify CS into ACTH-dependent (ACTH > 20 pg/mL) and ACTH-independent types (ACTH < 10 pg/mL).[2] Although very high levels of plasma ACTH (> 500 pg/mL) favor an ectopic source of ACTH production, the plasma ACTH alone cannot be relied upon to distinguish between a pituitary source (CD) and an ectopic source in ACTH-dependent CS. Tumors that may act as sources of ectopic ACTH production include carcinoid/neuroendocrine tumors, gastrinomas, medullary thyroid carcinoma, pheochromocytoma, bronchogenic

[a] Department of Neurological Surgery, University of Pittsburgh Medical Center, 200 Lothrop Street, Suite B-400, Pittsburgh, PA 15213-2582, USA
[b] Department of Radiology, University of Pittsburgh Medical Center, 200 Lothrop Street, Suite B-400, Pittsburgh, PA 15213-2582, USA
* Corresponding author. Department of Neurological Surgery, University of Pittsburgh Medical Center, 200 Lothrop Street, Suite B-400, Pittsburgh, PA 15213-258.
E-mail address: horowitzmb@upmc.edu (M.B. Horowitz).

Neurosurg Clin N Am 20 (2009) 361–367
doi:10.1016/j.nec.2009.01.003
1042-3680/09/$ – see front matter © 2009 Published by Elsevier Inc.

carcinoma, and pancreatic carcinoma.[3] The causes of CS are summarized in **Fig. 1**.

DIFFERENTIAL DIAGNOSIS OF CORTICOTROPIN-DEPENDENT CUSHING'S SYNDROME
Biochemical and Radiographic Testing

ACTH-dependent CS is defined as hypercortisolemia in the setting of normal or elevated levels of ACTH. The biochemical tests available for differentiating a pituitary source (CD) from an ectopic tumor include high-dose dexamethasone suppression testing (either 8-mg overnight or 2-day regimens), metyrapone stimulation, peripheral corticotropin-releasing hormone (CRH) stimulation, and desmopressin stimulation. These tests are founded on a central tenet that assumes ACTH-secreting pituitary tumors, unlike ectopic ACTH-secreting tumors, usually have partial responsiveness to suppression by elevated glucocorticoid levels and can be stimulated by either CRH or desmopressin.[4] These tests lack 100% accuracy, however. The high-dose dexamethasone suppression test remains in frequent use, but it has been shown to have low sensitivity (65%–100%) and specificity (60%–100%).[5] The peripheral CRH stimulation test has comparable sensitivity (70%–93%) and higher specificity (95%–100%) but is similarly unable to clinch the diagnosis of CD on its own.[6]

All patients suspected of having CD should undergo MRI of the brain with fine cuts through the sella turcica. Most ACTH-secreting pituitary tumors are intrasellar microadenomas (< 1 cm in diameter). Although MRI is an important adjunctive test in the differential diagnosis of ACTH-dependent CS, its utility is weakened by the high frequency of pituitary "incidentalomas" in the general population. Autopsy and radiographic studies have shown that pituitary microadenomas may be present in up to 20% of individuals.[7,8]

Moreover, the absence of a pituitary lesion on MRI does not rule out CD, because as many as 40% of patients who have CD have a negative MRI.[9] The introduction of the 3-Tesla MRI may help reduce the prevalence of CD patients who have a negative MRI, but experience with this stronger magnet currently is very limited.[10] Given that pituitary MRI often is equivocal in the setting of CD, only relatively large pituitary lesions (> 6 mm) on MRI in association with biochemically confirmed ACTH-dependent CS can safely clinch the diagnosis of CD.[11]

Bilateral Inferior Petrosal Sinus Sampling

BIPSS is a procedure in which ACTH levels are sampled from venous blood very near the pituitary gland and compared with peripheral blood ACTH levels to determine whether a pituitary tumor is the culprit for ACTH-dependent CS. In its unilateral form, inferior petrosal sinus (IPS) sampling was introduced in 1977 by Corrigan and colleagues[12] as a means of identifying the pituitary as the central cause of hypercortisolism. BIPSS was described by Doppman and colleagues[13] in 1984 and a year later by Oldfield and colleagues,[14] and Oldfield and colleagues reported on the use of BIPSS with and without the administration of CRH in the early 1990s.[15] There are numerous techniques for performing IPSS. The technique used at the University of Pittsburgh is described here (**Fig. 2**)[16]:

1. The patient is placed supine on the angiography suite table, and the right groin is prepped and draped in sterile fashion. Because BIPSS takes approximately 90 minutes; a Foley catheter is recommended for patient comfort.
2. The Seldinger technique is used to place two 5-F sheaths and one 4-F sheath into both common femoral veins. The authors prefer to

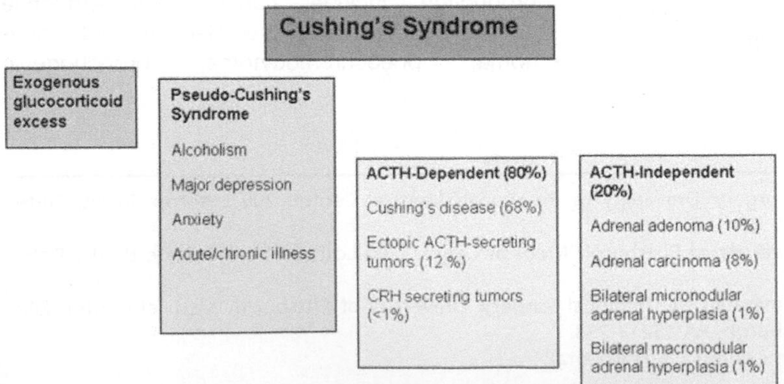

Cushing's Syndrome

Exogenous glucocorticoid excess	Pseudo-Cushing's Syndrome		
	Alcoholism		
	Major depression	**ACTH-Dependent (80%)**	**ACTH-Independent (20%)**
	Anxiety	Cushing's disease (68%)	Adrenal adenoma (10%)
	Acute/chronic illness	Ectopic ACTH-secreting tumors (12 %)	Adrenal carcinoma (8%)
		CRH secreting tumors (<1%)	Bilateral micronodular adrenal hyperplasia (1%)
			Bilateral macronodular adrenal hyperplasia (1%)

Fig. 1. Etiologies of Cushing's syndrome. (*From* Thomas AJ, Prevedello DM, Tomycz ND, et al. Diagnosis, perioperative care, and remission in Cushing's disease. Neurosurg Q 2008; 18(3):153–8.)

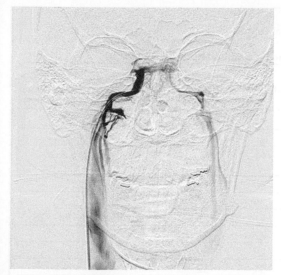

Fig. 2. Inferior petrosal sinus sampling. Anteroposterior view of venogram performed during BIPSS. Note catheter in the right IPS.

use one femoral vein for a 5-F and a 4-F sheath and the other for a 5-F sheath.
3. Through each 5-F sheath a straight 5-F catheter is advanced over a 0.038-inch hydrophilic wire with fluoroscopic guidance. One catheter is advanced into the right internal jugular vein (IJV), and the other is placed in the left IJV. Passage of endovascular catheters from the right atrium into the superior vena cava may engender transient cardiac ectopy. Gentle probing and wire manipulation may be necessary to advance a catheter into the left IJV, because a valve often is found at the junction between the left IJV and the left subclavian vein.
4. At the C1-2 level, the catheters and wires are carefully directed medially and anteriorly to access the IPS. Once an IPS is catheterized, venographic runs will opacify the ipsilateral IPS, superior petrosal sinus, cavernous sinus, and contralateral IPS. Roadmap guidance can help guide placement of the contralateral wire and catheter.
5. The authors prefer to use a 5-F catheter for sampling because the inner diameter permits rapid sampling of 5 to 10 cm^3 of blood at defined intervals. Moreover, they favor a straight catheter because they have found that angle-tipped catheters are easily occluded when the tip comes in contact with the venous wall during syringe aspiration.
6. The 4-F sheath is used for peripheral blood draws. Once the correct positioning of all catheters has been confirmed, blood sampling

commences under a protocol designed by endocrinologists at the University of Pittsburgh Medical Center (**Table 1**).
7. All catheters and sheaths are placed on continuous heparinized saline drips (6 units heparin/mL) to avoid catheter thrombosis. Before each sample is drawn, the catheters are aspirated, and saline-diluted blood is discarded.

When performing BIPSS via a femoral approach is not feasible because of aberrant anatomy or an inferior vena cava filter or thrombosis, direct IJV access is obtained. If an anastomosis between the IJV and IPS is missing, the 5-F catheters are placed at the C1-2 level for sampling. One should be aware, however, that sampling at this level may lead to false results secondary to transverse/sigmoid sinus contamination. Catheterization of the IPS is technically demanding, and even an experienced interventionalist may fail in up to 15% to 20% of cases.

ANATOMY OF BILATERAL INFERIOR PETROSAL SINUS SAMPLING

In most individuals, each IPS narrows to become a single vein that empties directly into the ipsilateral IJV, and in about 25% of individuals the IPS drainage forms a plexus of channels that empty into the IJV.[4] BIPSS is not possible in a small percentage of patients because there is no connection between the IPS and the IJV.[17] Approximately 60% of individuals exhibit symmetric pituitary venous drainage in which each half of the pituitary gland drains venous blood into the ipsilateral IPS.[18] This fact forms the basis for using BIPSS as a tool to lateralize corticotroph adenomas and makes bilateral sampling mandatory to avoid false-negative studies. One large series of 501 patients undergoing BIPSS attributed the 0.8% prevalence of false-negative results to a hypoplastic or anomalous IPS.[19] A classification system for IPS anatomic variants has been described.[20,21]

INTERPRETATION AND DIAGNOSTIC ACCURACY OF BILATERAL INFERIOR PETROSAL SINUS SAMPLING

ACTH secretion occurs in episodic bursts, and therefore the sensitivity of BIPSS can be increased by using CRH (1 mg/kg body weight) as a stimulating agent. In the absence of CRH, a central/peripheral ACTH value of 2.0 or greater strongly supports the diagnosis of CD.[15,22,23] Ovine CRH has been used primarily, but human-sequence CRH also has been shown to be an effective ACTH secretagogue.[24] A few studies have described augmenting CRH stimulation with

Table 1
The BIPSS protocol at the University of Pittsburgh Medical Center

Date:	Petrosal Venous Sampling with CRH Stimulation									
Sample	**Time Drawn**	**Right IPS ACTH**	**Left IPS ACTH**	**Peripheral ACTH**	**Peripheral CORTISOL**	**Right Jugular ACTH**	**Left Jugular ACTH**	**SVC ACTH**	**IVC Hepatic ACTH**	**IVC Renal ACTH**
−15 min		1	2	3	4					
−5 min		5	6	7						
0 (1.0 mcg/kg of CRH given)		8	9	10	11					
+2 min		12	13	14						
+5 min		15	16	17						
+10 min		18	19	20	21	22	23	24	25	26
+20 min					27	28				
+30 min					29	30				
+60 min					31	32				
+90 min					33	34				

All ACTH samples (Tubes 1–3, 5–7, 8–10, 12–14, 15–20, 22–26, 27, 29, 31, 33) are to be placed in purple top tubes and all Cortisol samples (Tubes 4, 11, 21, 28, 30, 32, 34) are placed in red top tubes. All tubes must be kept on ice until delivered to the lab. Tubes must also be numbered and labeled accordingly so that the lab cannot mix up the samples. This table is sent to the lab with all tubes at the end of the case for reference as to what time each sample is drawn.

(*From* Horowitz MB, Levy EI, Genevro J, et al. Petrosal sinus sampling for Cushing's disease. Prog Neurol Surg 2005; 17:232–8.)

desmopressin, but the value of this protocol has yet to be determined.[24–26] Following CRH stimulation, a central to peripheral ACTH ratio of 3.0 or greater highly favors the diagnosis of CD.[15,27] The current convention is that a positive BIPSS result represents a pituitary source, whereas a negative BIPSS result indicates an ectopic source.[4]

In a review of 21 studies that included a total of 569 patients, Newell-Price and colleagues[5] calculated that BIPSS with CRH stimulation had 96% sensitivity and 100% specificity in distinguishing CD from ectopic ACTH-dependent CS. Most studies to date have reported a 90% to 100% sensitivity and specificity for BIPSS.[26,28–31] A study by Swearingen and colleagues[32] found a lower specificity (67%) because half the patients in whom BIPSS suggested an ectopic source ultimately were found to have a pituitary tumor. Moreover, another study has shown that in about 15% of patients in whom BIPSS is positive for a central pituitary source, histologic confirmation of an adrenocorticotroph adenoma is missing.[33] The diagnostic accuracy of BIPSS has been shown to be superior to pituitary MRI and high-dose dexamethasone suppression testing.[34–36]

COMPLICATIONS OF BILATERAL INFERIOR PETROSAL SINUS SAMPLING

Serious complications after BIPSS are rare. Brainstem infarction, pontine hemorrhage, cranial nerve palsy, obstructive hydrocephalus, and venous subarachnoid hemorrhage have been reported.[37–42] Most centers (including the University of Pittsburgh Medical Center) have protocols involving bilateral simultaneous sampling of IPS blood; however, the concern that leaving catheters in situ within both IPSs may increase the risk of a brain stem insult has prompted some to favor sequential IPS sampling with immediate removal of catheters.[43] The mechanism of transient or permanent brainstem injury after BIPSS has been ascribed to either venous hypertension/outflow obstruction or impaired autoregulation leading to a form of posterior encephalopathy syndrome.[39] Other complications from BIPSS include deep venous thrombosis and pulmonary embolus for which prophylactic anticoagulation should be considered.[44,45]

LATERALIZATION WITH BILATERAL INFERIOR PETROSAL SINUS SAMPLING

Most patients who have CD have a pituitary microadenoma that is eccentric to one side of the pituitary and has venous drainage directly into the ipsilateral IPS.[44] This presentation forms the basis for using BIPSS as a lateralizing tool for ACTH-secreting pituitary tumors. Even when a pituitary source of ACTH secretion is confirmed by BIPSS, surgical exploration may fail to identify a pituitary adenoma. Knowledge of lateralization obtained beforehand may prompt the surgeon to perform a guided hemihypophysectomy. Unfortunately, BIPSS has proven to be a far superior diagnostic tool than a localizing tool. An interpetrosal gradient of 1.4 or more before or after CRH stimulation initially was proposed as a criterion for lateralization, and the reported accuracy was about 70%.[15] Incorrect lateralization from BIPSS has been attributed to asymmetric venous drainage with shunting of blood toward the dominant side; thus, some have insisted that venous angiography is necessary to judge the reliability of lateralizing data from BIPSS.[18] Although it is better than pituitary imaging, BIPSS has been shown to possess a wide range (50%–100%) of diagnostic accuracy for pituitary adenoma lateralization, and neurosurgeons must remain cautious about basing lateralizing operative decisions on BIPSS data alone.[5] The lateralizing ability of BIPSS may become particularly unreliable in patients who have had previous transsphenoidal surgery for CD.[27]

FALSE-NEGATIVE AND FALSE-POSITIVE RESULTS WITH BILATERAL INFERIOR PETROSAL SINUS SAMPLING

False-negative results after BIPSS have been explained by hypoplastic or plexiform IPS anatomy and by additional drainage from the pituitary into the portal sinuses ascending to the hypothalamus.[19,46] Dilution of venous blood by nonpituitary sources because of anastomosis between the IPS and the basilar venous plexus, retrograde drainage of the superior petrosal sinus, and misplaced catheters are other reported reasons for false-negative results during BIPSS.[47] There are fewer reports on false-positive results during BIPSS. One well-established reason for a false-positive result during BIPSS is the lack of hypercortisolism when the procedure is performed.[32,48,49] Hypercortisolemia is necessary during BIPSS to suppress normal corticotroph ACTH production, and medical treatment of hypercortisolism with drugs such as ketoconazole may compromise BIPSS. Before performing BIPSS, hypercortisolemia should be confirmed with a 24-hour urinary free cortisol or other test for hypercortisolism. False-positive results during BIPSS also may be caused by the rare entity of ectopic CRH production or by performing BIPSS in the setting of adrenal CS.[4] Finally, the importance of performing BIPSS only in the setting of established ACTH-dependent CS is highlighted by the fact that normal individuals as well as those who have pseudo-Cushing's states subjected to BIPSS have been shown to exhibit central to peripheral ACTH ratios similar to those seen in CD.[50] Thus, BIPSS can be potentially dangerous

and misleading when applied too early in the workup of CS, because a completely normal individual may be referred for surgical intervention, having been inappropriately diagnosed as having CD.

CAVERNOUS SINUS AND JUGULAR VENOUS SAMPLING

Jugular venous sampling has been proposed as a technically easier alternative to BIPSS, and such a strategy may be particularly suited for areas that lack the expertise or funding for BIPSS. One comparison study in 74 patients who had surgically confirmed CD showed that jugular venous sampling had specificity similar to that of BIPSS but a lower sensitivity (83% versus 94%).[29] Cavernous sinus sampling has been described as another alternative to BIPSS. The diagnostic accuracy of cavernous sinus sampling has not been shown to be superior to that of BIPSS, but some studies have suggested that sampling cavernous sinus blood, which is anatomically closer to the pituitary gland, may provide better lateralization data than BIPSS.[51–53] Because cavernous sinus sampling remains more technically challenging and may carry greater risk than BIPSS, further studies are needed to determine its role in the diagnostic evaluation of CD.

SUMMARY

Operative exploration aside, BIPSS remains the most powerful, albeit invasive, tool for the diagnosis of CD. BIPSS should be pursued in patients who meet the criteria of established ACTH-dependent CS with discordant imaging or biochemical tests and documented hypercortisolemia at the time of the procedure. Even so, BIPSS is not 100% accurate, and all diagnostic studies should be evaluated carefully by the multidisciplinary teams that manage CD. Although most research has focused on adults, BIPSS also has proven safe and effective as a differentiator between ectopic ACTH syndrome and CD in the pediatric population.[54] Future studies will investigate the potential of BIPSS to aid in the diagnosis of other pituitary disorders such as acromegaly.[55]

REFERENCES

1. Thomas AJ, Prevedello DM, Tomycz ND, et al. Diagnosis, perioperative care, and remission in Cushing's disease. Neurosurg Q 2008;18(3):153–8.
2. Arnaldi G, Angeli A, Atkinson AB, et al. Diagnosis and complications of Cushing's syndrome: a consensus statement. J Clin Endocrinol Metab 2003;88:5593–602.

3. Lad SP, Patil CG, Laws ER, et al. The role of inferior petrosal sinus sampling in the diagnostic localization of Cushing's disease. Neurosurg Focus 2007;23(3): E2.

4. Utz A, Biller BMK. The role of bilateral inferior petrosal sinus sampling in the diagnosis of Cushing's syndrome. Arq Bras Endocrinol Metabol 2007;51(8):1329–38.

5. Newell-Price J, Trainer P, Besser M, et al. The diagnosis and differential diagnosis of Cushing's syndrome and pseudo-Cushing's states. Endocr Rev 1998;19:647–72.

6. Lindsay J, Nieman L. Differential diagnosis and imaging in Cushing's syndrome. Endocrinol Metab Clin North Am 2005;34:4–3–421.

7. Molitch ME, Russell EJ. The pituitary "incidentaloma." An Int Med 1990;112(12):925–31.

8. Ezzat S, Asa SL, Couldwell WT, et al. The prevalence of pituitary adenomas: a systematic review. Cancer 2004;101:613–9.

9. Jagannathan J, Sheehan JP, Jane JA Jr. Evaluation and management of Cushing syndrome in case of negative sellar magnetic resonance imaging. Neurosurg Focus 2007;23(3):E3.

10. Kim LJ, Lekovic GP, White WL, et al. Preliminary experience with 3-Tesla MRI and Cushing's disease. Skull Base 2007;17(4):273–7.

11. Gross BA, Mindea SA, Pick AJ, et al. Diagnostic approach to Cushing disease. Neurosurg Focus 2007;23(3):E1.

12. Corrigan DF, Schaaf M, Whaley RA, et al. Selective venous sampling to differentiate ectopic ACTH secretion from pituitary Cushing's syndrome. N Engl J Med 1977;296:861–2.

13. Doppman JL, Oldfield EH, Krudy AG, et al. Petrosal sinus sampling of Cushing syndrome: anatomical and technical considerations. Radiology 1984;150: 99–103.

14. Oldfield EH, Girton ME, Doppman JL. Absence of intercavernous venous mixing: evidence supporting lateralization of pituitary microadenomas by venous sampling. J Clin Endocrinol Metab 1985;61:644–7.

15. Oldfield EH, Doppman JL, Nieman LK, et al. Petrosal sinus sampling with and without corticotropin-releasing hormone for the differential diagnosis of Cushing's syndrome. N Engl J Med 1991;325: 897–905.

16. Horowitz MB, Levy EI, Genevro J, et al. Petrosal sinus sampling for Cushing's disease. Prog Neurol Surg 2005;17:232–8.

17. Miller D, Doppman J. Petrosal sinus sampling: technique and rationale. Radiology 1991;178:37–47.

18. Mamelak A, Dowd C, Tyrrell J, et al. Venous angiography is needed to interpret inferior petrosal sinus and cavernous sinus sampling data for lateralizing adrenocorticotropin-secreting adenomas. J Clin Endocrinol Metab 1996;81:475–81.

19. Doppman JL, Chang R, Oldfield EH, et al. The hypoplastic inferior petrosal sinus: a potential source of false-negative results in petrosal sampling for Cushing's disease. J Clin Endocrinol Metab 1999;84:533–40.

20. Shiu PC, Hanafee WN, Wilson GH, et al. Cavernous sinus venography. AJR Am J Roentgenol 1968;104: 57–62.

21. Bonelli FS, Huston J, Carpenter PC, et al. Adrenocorticotropic hormone-dependent Cushing's syndrome: sensitivity and specificity of inferior petrosal sinus sampling. AJNR Am J Neuroradiol 2000;21:690–6.

22. Kai Y, Hamada J, Nishi T, et al. Usefulness of multiple-site venous sampling in the treatment of adrenocorticotropic hormone-producing pituitary adenoma. Surg Neurol 2003;59:292–9.

23. Pecori Giraldi F, Invitti C, Cavagnini F. Study Group of the Italian Society of Endocrinology and the Pathophysiology of the Hypothalamic-Pituitary-Adrenal Axis: the corticotropin-releasing hormone test in the diagnosis of ACTH-dependent Cushing's syndrome: a reappraisal. Clin Endocrinol (Oxf) 2001;54:601–7.

24. Kaltsas GA, Giannulis MG, Newell-Price JD, et al. A critical analysis of the value of simultaneous inferior petrosal sinus sampling in Cushing's disease and the occult ectopic adrenocorticotropin syndrome. J Clin Endocrinol Metab 1999;84(9):3401–2.

25. Tsagarakis S, Vassiliadi D, Kaskarelis IS, et al. The application of the combined corticotropin-releasing hormone plus desmopressin stimulation during petrosal sinus sampling is both sensitive and specific in differentiating patients with Cushing's disease from patients with the occult ectopic adrenocorticotropin syndrome. J Clin Endocrinol Metab 2007;92(6):2080–6.

26. Machado MC, de Sa SV, Domenice S, et al. The role of desmopressin in bilateral and simulataneous inferior petrosal sinus sampling for differential diagnosis of ACTH-dependent Cushing's syndrome. Clin Endocrinol (Oxf) 2007;66:136–42.

27. Lin L, Teng MM, Huang C, et al. Assessment of bilateral inferior petrosal sinus sampling (BIPSS) in the diagnosis of Cushing's disease. J Chin Med Assoc 2007;70(1):4–10.

28. Hernandez I, Espinosa-de-los-Monteros AL, Mendoza V, et al. Ectopic ACTH-secreting syndrome: a single center experience report with a high prevalence of occult tumor. Arch Med Res 2006;37:976–80.

29. Ilias I, Chang R, Pacak K, et al. Jugular venous sampling: an alternative to petrosal sinus sampling for the diagnostic evaluation of adrenocorticotropic hormone-dependent Cushing's syndrome. J Clin Endocrinol Metab 2004;89:3795–800.

30. Colao A, Faggiano A, Pivonello R, et al. Inferior petrosal sinus sampling in the differential diagnosis

of Cushing's syndrome: results of an Italian multi-center study. Eur J Endocrinol 2001;144:499–507.

31. Invitti C, Pecori Giraldi F, Cavagnini F. Inferior petrosal sinus sampling in patients with Cushing's syndrome and contradictory responses to dynamic testing. Clin Endocrinol (Oxf) 1999;51:255–7.

32. Swearingen B, Katznelson L, Miller K, et al. Diagnostic errors after inferior petrosal sinus sampling. J Clin Endocrinol Metab 2004;89:3752–63.

33. Locatelli M, Vance ML, Laws ER. Clinical review: the strategy of immediate reoperation for transsphenoidal surgery for Cushing's disease. J Clin Endocrinol Metab 2005;90:5478–82.

34. Midgette AS, Aron DC. High-dose dexamethasone suppression testing versus inferior petrosal sinus sampling in the differential diagnosis of adrenocorticotropin-dependent Cushing's syndrome: a decision analysis. Am J Med Sci 1995;309(3):162–70.

35. Booth GL, Redelmeier DA, Grosman H, et al. Improved diagnostic accuracy of inferior petrosal sinus sampling over imaging for localizing pituitary pathology in patients with Cushing's disease. J Clin Endocrinol Metab 1998;83(7):2291–5.

36. Wiggam MI, Heaney AP, McIlrath EM, et al. Bilateral inferior petrosal sinus sampling in the differential diagnosis of adrenocorticotropin-dependent Cushing's syndrome: a comparison with other diagnostic tests. J Clin Endocrinol Metab 2000;85(4):1525–32.

37. Bonelli FS, Huston J 3rd, Meyer FB, et al. Venous subarachnoid hemorrhage after inferior petrosal sinus sampling for adrenocorticotropic hormone. AJNR Am J Neuroradiol 1999;20(2):306–7.

38. Miller DL, Doppman JK, Peterman SB, et al. Neurologic complications of petrosal sinus sampling. Radiology 1992;185:143–7.

39. Gandhi CD, Meyer SA, Patel AB. Neurologic complications of inferior petrosal sinus sampling. AJNR Am J Neuroradiol 2008;29:760–5.

40. Sturrock ND, Jeffcoate WJ. A neurological complication of inferior petrosal sinus sampling during investigation for Cushing's disease: a case report. J Neurol Neurosurg Psychiatr 1997;62:527–8.

41. Seyer H, Honegger J, Schott W, et al. Raymond's syndrome following petrosal sinus sampling. Acta Neurochir (Wien) 1994;131:157–9.

42. Lefournier V, Gatta B, Martinie M, et al. One transient neurological complication (sixth nerve palsy) in 166 consecutive inferior petrosal sinus samplings for the etiological diagnosis of Cushing's syndrome. J Clin Endocrinol Metab 1999;84:3401–2.

43. Padayatty SJ, Orme SM, Nelson M, et al. Bilateral sequential inferior petrosal sinus sampling with corticotropin-releasing hormone stimulation in the

44. Obuobie J, Davies JS, Ogunko A, et al. Venous thrombo-embolism following inferior petrosal sinus sampling in Cushing's disease. J Endocrinol Invest 2000;23(8):542–4.

45. Oldfield EH, Chrousos GP, Schulte HM, et al. Preoperative lateralization of ACTH-secreting pituitary microadenomas by bilateral and simultaneous inferior petrosal sinus sampling. N Engl J Med 1985;312:100–3.

46. Bergland RM, Page RB. Can the pituitary secrete directly to the brain? (affirmative anatomical evidence). Endocrinology 1978;102:1325–38.

47. Doppman JL, Krudy AG, Girton ME, et al. Basilar venous plexus of the posterior fossa: a potential source of error in petrosal sinus sampling. Radiology 1985;155:375–8.

48. Burman P, Lethagen A, Ivancev K, et al. Dual bronchial carcinoids and Cushing's syndrome with a paradoxical response to dexamethasone and a false positive outcome of inferior petrosal sinus sampling. Eur J Endocrinol 2008;159:483–8.

49. Yamamoto Y, Davis DH, Todd B, et al. False-positive petrosal sinus sampling in the diagnosis of Cushing's disease. Report of two cases. J Neurosurg 1995;83:1087–91.

50. Yanovski J, Cutler G Jr, Doppman J, et al. The limited ability of inferior petrosal sinus sampling with corticotropin-releasing hormone to distinguish Cushing's disease from pseudo-Cushing states or normal physiology. J Clin Endocrinol Metab 1993;77:503–9.

51. Liu C, Lo JC, Dowd CF, et al. Cavernous and inferior petrosal sinus sampling in the evaluation of ACTH-dependent Cushing's syndrome. Clin Endocrinol (Oxf) 2004;61(4):478–86.

52. Fujimura M, Ikeda H, Takahashi A, et al. Diagnostic value of super-selective bilateral cavernous sinus sampling with hypothalamic stimulating hormone loading in patients with ACTH-producing pituitary adenoma. Neurol Res 2005;27:11–5.

53. Gazioglu N, Ulu MO, Ozlen F, et al. Management of Cushing's disease using cavernous sinus sampling: effectiveness in tumor lateralization. Clin Neurol Neurosurg 2008;110(4):333–8.

54. Lienhardt A, Grossman AB, Dacie JE, et al. Relative contributions of inferior petrosal sinus sampling and pituitary imaging in the investigation of children and adolescents with ACTH-dependent Cushing's syndrome. J Clin Endocrinol Metab 2001;86(12):5711–4.

55. Doppman JL, Miller DL, Patronas NJ, et al. The diagnosis of acromegaly: value of inferior petrosal sinus sampling. AJR Am J Roentgenol 1990;154(5):1075–7.

diagnosis of Cushing's disease. Eur J Endocrinol 1998;139:161–6.

Intracranial Endovascular Balloon Test Occlusion— Indications, Methods, and Predictive Value

N. Chaudhary[a], J. J. Gemmete[a],
B. G. Thompson, MD[b], A. S. Pandey[b],*

KEYWORDS

- Endovascular • Neuroimaging
- Balloon test occlusion • Presurgical testing
- Brain surgery

The evolution of endovascular technology has allowed the treatment of complex vascular pathologies. Although advances in stent and coil technology are at the heart of this treatment, parent vessel occlusion remains an important method of treating pathologies that are not amenable to other technologies. Endovascular parent vessel occlusion with detachable balloons dates back to the early 1970s and was first reported by Serbinenko.[1,2]

Wide-necked giant aneurysms, pseudoaneurysms, traumatic vascular injuries, carotid blowout injuries, and carotid fistulas are examples of conditions that require parent vessel obliteration as a treatment modality. Patients harboring head and neck cancers also may require permanent carotid artery occlusion as preoperative preparation for tumor resection. The efficacy and necessity of such treatment is evident, but avoiding immediate or delayed cerebral ischemia remains a challenge.

The main complication associated with permanent vessel occlusion (PBO) is related to ischemic changes from hypoperfusion or thromboembolic phenomenon. (In this article, permanent vessel occlusion is referred to as "PBO" even though balloons are no longer used to occlude vessels.)

Linskey and colleagues[3] reported that PBO in 254 patients without balloon test occlusion (BTO) led to a high ischemic complication rate: 26% of patients suffered infarcts with a 12% mortality. Although embolic complications are treated with anticoagulation, a hypoperfusion state is best treated by choosing patients who will not develop such a state. The BTO is one method by which surgeons evaluate whether a patient will be able to tolerate permanent occlusion of an extracranial or intracranial vessel. Those who fail such an evaluation require revascularization procedures before parent vessel occlusion. This article discusses the indications, methods, predictive value, and complications of the BTO. It also briefly describes the Wada test in the context of preoperative evaluation of patients who are candidates for temporal lobectomy.

TECHNIQUES FOR BALLOON TEST OCCLUSION

Although there are several techniques for performing the BTO procedure, the underlying principle is to assess the efficacy of the collateral circulation in maintaining perfusion of the affected vascular territories. Clinical tolerance of permanent occlusion of a vessel can be assessed by a number of

[a] Department of Radiology/Neuroradiology, University of Michigan Hospitals, Ann Arbor, MI, USA
[b] Department of Neurosurgery, University of Michigan, Ann Arbor, MI, USA
* Corresponding author.
E-mail address: adityap@med.umich.edu (A.S. Pandey).

Neurosurg Clin N Am 20 (2009) 369–375
doi:10.1016/j.nec.2009.01.004
1042-3680/09/$ – see front matter © 2009 Published by Elsevier Inc.

objective evaluations: clinical examination, neuro-physiologic monitoring, perfusion scanning, or angiographic assessment. Most centers use several of these methods to assess the clinical safety of PBO.

Standard Technique

Informed consent is obtained from all patients in the presence of family members (if applicable). When clinical examination is to be assessed, patients are awake, and the procedure is performed under local anesthetic. Benzodiazepines should not be used, because they can interfere with memory functions and related tasks. Patients are told that they will be asked questions evaluating their memory, speech, motor, sensory, and analytical skills (calculations) while the procedure is being performed. In addition, patients should be warned that contrast administration during the procedure could lead to abnormal sensations within the face region.

A 6-F femoral sheath then is introduced into the femoral artery using a single-wall puncture technique. Although either femoral artery can be used, the authors try to puncture the femoral artery opposite the side of pathology. This precaution ensures that any complication associated with the TBO, PBO, or placement of the femoral sheath will only affect one extremity. A baseline activated clotting time (ACT) is drawn, and the patient is given 70 U/kg of heparin. ACT is assessed at 5 minutes after heparinization and then every 15 minutes as needed. The goal ACT is approximately two times baseline to prevent procedure-related thromboembolic complications.

A 5-F diagnostic catheter then is used to perform four-vessel cerebral and cervical angiography in the anteroposterior and lateral projections. A 6-F guide catheter is introduced into the common carotid artery. A nondetachable balloon catheter then is introduced and positioned in the high cervical segment of the internal carotid artery. Any lower positioning of the balloon can cause a carotid sinus reflex leading to significant bradycardia. This complication is the main reason BTO procedures are not performed from the common carotid artery: doing so leads to a decreased pressure within the carotid sinus that reflexively causes an increase in arterial blood pressure. Such a reflex can give false clinical results, because the arterial blood pressure could be much lower in a normal state. Although the authors have not experienced significant alterations in arterial blood pressure or heart rate during BTO procedures, they always are prepared with temporary pacing wires and atropine should the situation arise.

The balloon is inflated with angiographic confirmation of complete occlusion of the vessel in question. Neurologic examination then is performed by the operating surgeon for a total duration of 30 minutes. It is important to encourage the patient to report any change in sensory function, such as visual deterioration. If there are any changes in the patient's neurologic state, the balloon is deflated immediately, and cerebral angiography is performed.

After this evaluation the balloon is deflated, and an angiogram is performed to ensure normal patency of the vessel and its distal territory. There is continuous 12-lead electroencephalogram (EEG) monitoring as well. Then the catheters are removed, and hemostasis at the groin puncture is secured by manual compression. If the patient does not develop any neurologic symptoms during this time, the assessment is that the parent vessel can be completely occluded. Before discharge, the patient is observed for 4 hours with neurologic evaluation every 15 minutes.

Modifications to the Basic Technique

Venous-phase assessment: predictive value of balloon test occlusion tolerance

Venous-phase comparison of the two hemispheres certainly can evaluate the presence and functionality of the collateral circulation. It has been assumed that patients who have symmetry within the venous phase during BTO harbor enough collateral circulation to tolerate a PBO procedure. This comparison can be accomplished easily by performing angiography through the vertebral and contralateral internal carotid artery (ICA) while the balloon is inflated. This hypothesis has been tested by Abud and colleagues[3] and van Rooij and colleagues.[4] These investigators performed angiographic assessment as well as clinical evaluation during BTO procedures. The angiographic assessment compared the venous phase in the hemispheres or in supratentorial and infratentorial structures, depending on whether the collateral flow was from the anterior communicating artery or the posterior communicating artery. A delay of more than 0.5 milliseconds was considered to indicate high ischemic risk for PBO. Of the 49 surviving patients in this series who had passed the angiographic evaluation and had undergone PBO, one patient developed a delayed ischemic event, thus giving this evaluation a positive predictive value of 98%.

Abud and colleagues[3] also tested this hypothesis in reporting on 60 patients who had undergone a PBO procedure. In all these patients the venous state had been evaluated angiographically during the BTO procedure. These patients were not tested clinically, because the procedure was performed under general anesthesia. A delay of more than 2 seconds within the venous phase of the hemispheres was considered a failed test. Fifty-seven of the 60 patients had a delay of less than 2 seconds, and none of these patients suffered any ischemic complications post PBO. Of the three patients who had a delay greater than 2 seconds, one suffered an ischemic complication.[3] Most certainly the predictive value of this technique is powerful; however, this procedure requires bilateral femoral artery catheterization and further catheterization of the cervical vasculature. Although both these series were free of periprocedural complications, this method certainly requires further intravascular manipulation, theoretically increasing the probability of vessel dissection or emboli.

Measurement of stump pressures

Arterial pressure can be monitored by a double-lumen catheter positioned distal to the occlusion site with the second lumen connected to a pressure transducer. Morishima and colleagues[5] have reported that maintenance of a stump pressure ratio (initial mean stump pressure/preocclusion mean arterial pressure) of 60% or more during BTO is a useful marker of adequate collateral circulation. The utility of this technique is controversial, because, although a number of studies have found a significant correlation between stump pressures and measures of cerebral perfusion, such as single-proton emission CT (SPECT),[6] others have not.[7]

Induced hypotension

Collateral circulation can be challenged further by inducing hypotension during a BTO procedure. Dare and colleagues[8] studied 13 patients undergoing BTO with a hypotensive challenge. This challenge is applied in patients who have tolerated 15 to 20 minutes of arterial occlusion while normotensive. The mean arterial pressure typically is lowered by 30% of baseline (using intravenous nitroprusside or labetalol) and is maintained for an additional 15 to 20 minutes with continued clinical evaluation. Using this technique Standard and colleagues[9] demonstrated identified an additional 19% of patients who had limited collateral circulation; the false-negative rate was 5%. Dare and colleagues,[8] however, reported a false-negative rate of 15%. They suggest that the vasodilatory effect on the cerebral circulation caused by the direct pharmacologic effect of nitroprusside increases the false-negative rate. Overall the literature does not show that a hypotensive challenge is superior to a traditional BTO.

Balloon test occlusion and perfusion assessment

Single-photon emission computed tomography Tc-99m hexamethylpropylene-amine oxime (HMPAO) is the tracer injected approximately 2 minutes after the BTO. A study typically is done 1 to 6 hours later. The sensitivity of this type of imaging is very high, but the specificity is poor. In one study all patients who had focal defects on SPECT immediately after occlusion test returned to normal at repeat SPECT examination at 24 hours.[10] There also are reports of use of [15O]H_2O positron emission tomography for quantitative measurements of cerebral blood flow (CBF) during BTO.[11] This test is performed during BTO and then after the deflation of the balloon.

CT perfusion with acetazolamide challenge CT perfusion before and after the injection of acetazolamide also has been reported as an adjunct to BTO. While undergoing BTO, patients are transferred to the CT suite for CT perfusion scanning with the administration of acetazolamide.[12] Acetazolamide penetrates the blood–brain barrier slowly by diffusion and inhibits carbonic anhydrase, thus causing acidosis. This increase in acidity leads to compensatory dilation of small arterioles. It is thought that the increase in CBF induced by acetazolamide is reduced if compensatory vasodilation associated with a decrease in CBF from BTO already has occurred.[13] This procedure, however, involves the transfer of the patient to the CT suite with a balloon in place within the carotid, thus increasing the probability of injury to the vessel.

Xenon CT perfusion Xenon CT perfusion is another modality to quantify CBF in patients who have clinically tolerated a test occlusion.[14–16] The patient inhales a gas mixture of 33% xenon and 67% oxygen. Scans are performed as baseline before balloon occlusion and then are repeated during balloon inflation. Xenon uptake in the middle cerebral artery territory is used to estimate regional CBF with the threshold for predicting delayed ischemic stroke set at less than 30 mL/100 g/min.

MR perfusion MR perfusion imaging with dynamic gadolinium enhancement can be performed during BTO when MR is available in the angiography suite.[2] A bolus injection of gadolinium is administered at dose of 0.1 mmol/kg, and various parameters such as cerebral blood volume, mean transit time, and regional CBF can be calculated.

In patients who have clinically failed test occlusion, authors have demonstrated greater perfusion delays and asymmetry in contrast enhancement and in parenchymal signal intensity in the areas of hypoperfusion.

Transcranial Doppler ultrasound The use of transcranial Doppler (TCD) ultrasound to evaluate flow in the middle cerebral artery is well documented in the literature. This technique can be used as an adjunct in the evaluation of collateral flow in BTO procedures. TCD has the advantage of being noninvasive; but the correlation between CBF and mean velocity in the middle cerebral artery is not a direct one, because vessel caliber, hematocrit, and viscosity affect the velocity in the blood vessel.[15] Eckert and colleagues[17] recommend that a reduction in mean blood flow velocity and pulsatility index of less than 30% is a good predictor of clinical tolerance of occlusion, whereas a reduction of these values by more than 50% indicates failure of the BTO.

Neurophysiologic monitoring The use of neurophysiologic monitoring (NPM) (ie, short-latency somatosensory-evoked potential [SSEP], EEG, and brain stem–evoked potentials) is well documented as an important adjunct in endovascular treatment modalities. NPM certainly is of value when clinical assessment cannot be performed (eg, in a patient under general anesthesia). A regional CBF of 15 mL/100 g/min seems to be a critical value below which cortical SSEP amplitude is reduced, central conduction time is prolonged, and cerebral infarction is likely to occur. Liu and colleagues[18] claim that although this technique has limitations, treatment decisions were altered because of NPM for 5 patients in their series of 35 patients; hence they believe NPM is a useful adjunct to clinical neurologic testing during BTO.

DISCUSSION

Despite the innovative technological advances in endovascular neurosurgery, parent vessel occlusion remains an important modality in the treatment of complex vascular pathologies. Sudden ligation of the ICA is not ideal, because it leads to a significant risk of ischemic stroke. Linskey and colleagues[16] have quoted a 26% risk of ischemia with abrupt ICA occlusion, as compared with a 13% risk when BTO was used before permanent occlusion. Many techniques (NPM, hypotensive challenge, venous-phase evaluation, and perfusion measurements) have been evaluated as adjuncts to a clinical BTO evaluation to enhance the predictive value of a successful BTO.[8,11,19–22]

Ischemic complications in patients undergoing PBO result from either thromboembolism or hypoperfusion. Although anticoagulation can decrease the incidence of embolic complications, hypoperfusion is best treated with a cerebral bypass procedure. The goal of BTO procedures is to identify the individuals who would benefit from cerebral bypass before PBO and thereby reduce the risk of hypoperfusion-related complications.

In essence, a BTO procedure evaluates the efficacy of the collateral circulation. Primary collaterals are those that relate to the circle of Willis (the anterior communicating artery and the posterior communicating artery). The secondary collaterals consist of retrograde flow within the ophthalmic artery, external carotid feeders, and leptomeningeal collaterals. The presence of primary collaterals, especially the anterior communicating artery complex, leads to a decrease in the incidence and volume of internal zone infarcts (corona radiate, centrum semiovale), as reported by Bisschops and colleagues. Although the efficacy of primary collaterals is tested with a BTO, secondary collaterals are difficult to evaluate, because they can take months to develop. Rutgers and colleagues[23] have shown that secondary collaterals are more important than primary collaterals. They followed 62 patients who had a symptomatic ICA occlusion but who remained asymptomatic over a 2-year span. During this time, there was no change in flow directionality across the anterior communicating artery and posterior communicating artery, and the flow within the ophthalmic artery became antegrade. Thus leptomeningeal collaterals must have prevented hypoperfusion-related complications.

The use of various adjunctive techniques and combinations of these techniques certainly has lessened the ischemic risks associated with hypoperfusion. Comparison of the venous filling phase between the occluded and the normal contralateral side seems to be the most useful evaluation.[3] This evaluation can be performed with or without a clinical examination and lasts for 20 to 30 minutes. (If done without a clinical evaluation, the procedure can be shortened, because only angiographic data are evaluated.) In the retrospective study of 60 patients, 57 had an uneventful outcome from permanent occlusion, accurately predicted by the venous-phase delay of 2 seconds or less. Of the three patients who had a delay of more than 3 seconds, one developed watershed area infarction without clinical sequelae. This technique needs to be studied as a part of a larger prospective trial to verify its positive predictive value and long-term outcome.

Angiographic description and quantification of cross flow were found to have no predictive value for tolerance of ICA occlusion, nor could the presence of cerebral ischemia be associated with specific patterns of flow within the circle of Willis.[24,25] The same was true for hypotensive challenge, which failed to improve long-term outcome of patients undergoing PBO. The patients identified by a trial occlusion test with additional neurophysiologic monitoring were similar to those identified by clinical surveillance alone.[16] The addition of a stable xenon-enhanced CT reduced postoperative infarction and mortality rates only insignificantly compared with clinical temporary test occlusion alone.[16] Additionally, xenon inhalation has adverse reactions such as patient motion, spontaneous respiratory depression, and induction of rapid changes in CBF itself.[16,26-28] The CT perfusion method described is cumbersome and sophisticated, involving the transfer of a patient to the CT suite with a balloon catheter in the carotid. These measures certainly add to the risk of the investigation. The other method of xenon-enhanced CT has similar limitations. The HMPAO SPECT technique requires 24 to 48 hours before results can be obtained; a repeat examination within this time period is required because of the half-life of this isotope. The TCD method is a user-friendly and convenient adjunct but needs trained personnel and provides no further improvement in outcome.[27]

FUTURE

BTO performed with clinical assessment is a powerful tool for assessing a patient's ability to tolerate a PBO procedure. The technological advance of perfusion measurement by multidetector CT (eg, the 320-slice Aquilion from Toshiba) is an important adjunct during BTO procedures. Angiographic evaluation with the comparison of venous phases shows great promise but will require further validation with a larger study. This technique can be performed under general anesthesia and thus is more comfortable for the patient; it also is a shorter procedure. In addition, the PBO can be performed immediately following the TBO, because the patient already is under general anesthesia and is anticoagulated.

THE WADA TEST

The intracarotid amobarbital test injection is performed in conjunction with neuropsychological testing to determine lateralization of speech/language and memory functions. In the majority of cases it is performed in patients with medically intractable epilepsy scheduled for surgical resection of epileptogenic tissue; however, it is also employed for non-epileptic patients scheduled for resection of unilateral temporal or frontotemporal lesions.[26,27,30]

The procedure was first performed by Juhn A. Wada using amobarbital in the 1940s to arrest convulsions in patients with status epilepticus. He first described the use of this procedure to determine language lateralization in 1949.[26] He introduced the Amytal test to the Montreal Neurological Institute in 1955. This led to rapid worldwide use reflecting its importance in preventing surgical cognitive deficits.[34] In 1960, he collaborated with Rasmussen to report the use of this test to determine hemispheric language dominance in patients for epilepsy surgery.

TECHNIQUE

The procedure is performed under a local anesthetic to facilitate neuropsychological testing during the exam. The cerebral hemisphere harboring the presumed lesion is studied first by angiography. After angiography, a hand directed injection of sodium Amytal is given. The dose typically ranges from 75 to 130 mg. The dose administered by the left and right injections is identical. Following the injection and during the period of maximal drug effect, language and verbal memory are studied.[6] The contra lateral carotid is selected to repeat the procedure after allowing for a period of 30–45 minutes for the effects of the amobarbital to settle down from the previous injection. It is recommended to use a microcatheter in a more selective location if there are normal variant anastomoses between the carotid and the basilar vasculature or when there is significant crossflow through the anterior communicating artery. This can result in bifrontal impairment that can render the neuropsychological testing invalid due to impaired patient consciousness and inability to cooperate. The selective middle and posterior cerebral artery position has been suggested with reduced doses of the agent (75–80 mg).

DISCUSSION

While the WDA test is useful in language localization, a recent survey conducted around the world (USA, Europe, Asia, Australia & Canada – 92 epilepsy centers in 32 countries) suggests that there has been a decrease in the use of Wada procedures for presurgical evaluation of surgery candidates over the past 15 years (85% to 12% since 1993).[3] Such a drop in usage of the WADA testing correlates with the arrival of non-invasive cortical functionality testing. It has been argued that the Amytal test mimics the effects of surgery better, because most of the alternatives include activation instead of inactivation paradigms. Advances in non-invasive inactivation procedures, such as transcranial magnetic stimulation, may silence this criticism in the future. Additionally, magneto encephalography and functional magnetic resonance imaging may provide better localizing information.

It is established that invasive amytal test has its own risks as of any diagnostic catheter cerebral angiography. It can confound the circumstances in which neuropsychological testing is performed and can deselect patients from potentially curative surgery for intractable epilepsy by a false positive result. If reliable information can be obtained from non invasive methods like functional MRI then the practice of epilepsy surgery evaluation may move towards such. The drawback of the modern day non-invasive functional imaging is that it is not yet widely available or accessible.

In words of Juhn A. Wada, as he had expressed 11 years back, "while we await the arrival of validated safe alternative(s), judicious and innovative use of carotid amytal deactivation by a skilled hand, when justified, cannot only continue to help patients but also create new information and hypotheses on the mechanism of function and dysfunction of the human brain in the behavioral state."[34] A recent study has shown that a systematic study of MR imaging-acquired morphological data and Wada-acquired neuropsychological data may increase our understanding of the location of material-specific memory and the selection of eligible candidates for epilepsy surgery.[6] The WADA test remains a valuable preoperative tool in evaluating language localization.

REFERENCES

1. Serbinenko FA. [Catheterization and occlusion of major cerebral vessels and prospects for the development of vascular neurosurgery]. Vopr Neirokhir 1971;35:17–27.

2. Serbinenko FA. Balloon catheterization and occlusion of major cerebral vessels. J Neurosurg 1974; 41:125–45.

3. Abud DG, Spelle L, Piotin M, et al. Venous phase timing during balloon test occlusion as a criterion for permanent internal carotid artery sacrifice. AJNR Am J Neuroradiol 2005;26:2602–9.

4. van Rooij WJ, Sluzewski M, Metz NH, et al. Carotid balloon occlusion for large and giant aneurysms: evaluation of a new test occlusion protocol. Neurosurgery 2000;47:116–21 [discussion: 122].

5. Morishima H, Kurata A, Miyasaka Y, et al. Efficacy of the stump pressure ratio as a guide to the safety of permanent occlusion of the internal carotid artery. Neurol Res 1998;20:732–6.

6. Tomura N, Omachi K, Takahashi S, et al. Comparison of technetium Tc 99m hexamethylpropyleneamine oxime single-photon emission tomograph with stump pressure during the balloon occlusion test of the internal carotid artery. AJNR Am J Neuroradiol 2005;26:1937–42.

7. Barker DW, Jungreis CA, Horton JA, et al. Balloon test occlusion of the internal carotid artery: change in stump pressure over 15 minutes and its correlation with xenon CT cerebral blood flow. AJNR Am J Neuroradiol 1993;14:587–90.

8. Dare AO, Chaloupka JC, Putman CM, et al. Failure of the hypotensive provocative test during temporary balloon test occlusion of the internal carotid artery to predict delayed hemodynamic ischemia after therapeutic carotid occlusion. Surg Neurol 1998; 50:147–55 [discussion: 146–5].

9. Standard SC, Ahuja A, Guterman LR, et al. Balloon test occlusion of the internal carotid artery with hypotensive challenge. AJNR Am J Neuroradiol 1995;16: 1453–8.

10. Simonson TM, Ryals TJ, Yuh WT, et al. MR imaging and HMPAO scintigraphy in conjunction with balloon test occlusion: value in predicting sequelae after permanent carotid occlusion. AJR Am J Roentgenol 1992;159:1063–8.

11. Brunberg JA, Frey KA, Horton JA, et al. [15O]H2O positron emission tomography determination of cerebral blood flow during balloon test occlusion of the internal carotid artery. AJNR Am J Neuroradiol 1994;15:725–32.

12. Jain R, Hoeffner EG, Deveikis JP, et al. Carotid perfusion CT with balloon occlusion and acetazolamide challenge test: feasibility. Radiology 2004;231:906–13.

13. Okudaira Y, Arai H, Sato K. Cerebral blood flow alteration by acetazolamide during carotid balloon occlusion: parameters reflecting cerebral perfusion pressure in the acetazolamide test. Stroke 1996; 27:617–21.

14. Johnson DW, Stringer WA, Marks MP, et al. Stable xenon CT cerebral blood flow imaging: rationale for and role in clinical decision making. AJNR Am J Neuroradiol 1991;12:201–13.

15. Kofke WA, Brauer P, Policare R, et al. Middle cerebral artery blood flow velocity and stable xenon-enhanced computed tomographic blood flow during balloon test occlusion of the internal carotid artery. Stroke 1995;26:1603–6.

16. Linskey ME, Jungreis CA, Yonas H, et al. Stroke risk after abrupt internal carotid artery sacrifice: accuracy of preoperative assessment with balloon test occlusion and stable xenon-enhanced CT. AJNR Am J Neuroradiol 1994;15:829–43.

17. Eckert B, Thie A, Carvajal M, et al. Predicting hemo-dynamic ischemia by transcranial Doppler moni-toring during therapeutic balloon occlusion of the internal carotid artery. AJNR Am J Neuroradiol 1998;19:577–82.

18. Liu AY, Lopez JR, Do HM, et al. Neurophysiological monitoring in the endovascular therapy of aneu-rysms. AJNR Am J Neuroradiol 2003;24:1520–7.

19. Eskridge JM. Xenon-enhanced CT: past and present. AJNR Am J Neuroradiol 1994;15:845–6.

20. Michel E, Liu H, Remley KB, et al. Perfusion MR neu-roimaging in patients undergoing balloon test occlu-sion of the internal carotid artery. AJNR Am J Neuroradiol 2001;22:1590–6.

21. van der Schaaf IC, Brilstra EH, Buskens E, et al. En-dovascular treatment of aneurysms in the cavernous sinus: a systematic review on balloon occlusion of the parent vessel and embolization with coils. Stroke 2002;33:313–8.

22. Vazquez Anon V, Aymard A, Gobin YP, et al. Balloon occlusion of the internal carotid artery in 40 cases of giant intracavernous aneurysm: technical aspects, cerebral monitoring, and results. Neuroradiology 1992;34:245–51.

23. Rutgers DR, Klijn CJ, Kappelle LJ, et al. A longitu-dinal study of collateral flow patterns in the circle of Willis and the ophthalmic artery in patients with a symptomatic internal carotid artery occlusion. Stroke 2000;31:1913–20.

24. Beatty RA, Richardson AE. Predicting intolerance to common carotid artery ligation by carotid angiog-raphy. J Neurosurg 1968;28:9–13.

25. Jawad K, Miller D, Wyper DJ, et al. Measurement of CBF and carotid artery pressure compared with cerebral angiography in assessing collateral blood supply after carotid ligation. J Neurosurg 1977;46:185–96.

26. Giller CA, Mathews D, Walker B, et al. Prediction of tolerance to carotid artery occlusion using transcra-nial Doppler ultrasound. J Neurosurg 1994;81:15–9.

27. Giller CA, Purdy P, Lindstrom WW. Effects of inhaled stable xenon on cerebral blood flow velocity. AJNR Am J Neuroradiol 1990;11:177–82.

28. Latchaw RE, Yonas H, Pentheny SL, et al. Adverse reactions to xenon-enhanced CT cerebral blood flow determination. Radiology 1987;163:251–4.

29. Snyder PJ, Harris LJ. The intracarotid amobarbital procedure: an historical perspective. Brain Cogn 1997;33:18–32.

30. Spencer DC, Morrell MJ, Risinger MW. The role of the intracarotid amobarbital procedure in evaluation of patients for epilepsy surgery. Epilepsia 2000;41:320–5.

31. Trenerry MR, Loring DW. Intracarotid amobarbital procedure. The Wada test. Neuroimaging Clin N Am 1995;5:721–8.

32. Wada JA. A fateful encounter: sixty years later–reflec-tions on the Wada test. Epilepsia 2008;49:726–7.

33. Cohen-Gadol AA, Westerveld M, Alvarez-Carilles J, et al. Intracarotid Amytal memory test and hippo-campal magnetic resonance imaging volumetry: val-idity of the Wada test as an indicator of hippocampal integrity among candidates for epilepsy surgery. J Neurosurg 2004;101:926–31.

34. Baxendale S, Thompson PJ, Duncan JS. The role of the Wada test in the surgical treatment of temporal lobe epilepsy: an international survey. Epilepsia 2008;49:715–20.

Index

Note: Page numbers of article titles are in **boldface** type.

Neurosurg Clin N Am 20 (2009) 377–382
doi:10.1016/S1042-3680(09)00062-X
1042-3680/09/$ – see front matter © 2009 Elsevier Inc. All rights reserved

Moving?

Make sure your subscription moves with you!

To notify us of your new address, find your **Clinics Account Number** (located on your mailing label above your name), and contact customer service at:

Email: journalscustomerservice-usa@elsevier.com

800-654-2452 (subscribers in the U.S. & Canada)
314-447-8871 (subscribers outside of the U.S. & Canada)

Fax number: 314-447-8029

Elsevier Health Sciences Division
Subscription Customer Service
3251 Riverport Lane
Maryland Heights, MO 63043

*To ensure uninterrupted delivery of your subscription, please notify us at least 4 weeks in advance of move.

Moving?

Make sure your subscription moves with you!

To notify us of your new address, find your Clinics Account Number (located on your mailing label above your name) and contact customer service at:

Email: journalscustomerservice-usa@elsevier.com

800-654-2452 (subscribers in the U.S. & Canada)
314-447-8871 (subscribers outside of the U.S. & Canada)

Fax number: 314-447-8029

Elsevier Health Sciences Division
Subscription Customer Service
3251 Riverport Lane
Maryland Heights, MO 63043

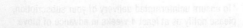

Printed and bound by CPI Group (UK) Ltd, Croydon, CR0 4YY

OAHO10264

0-HN0365-0027

Printed and bound by CPI Group (UK) Ltd, Croydon, CR0 4YY

03/10/2024

01040362-0002